D0927904

Bowls of Goodness

Vibrant Vegetarian Recipes
Full of Nourishment

Recipes and Photography by

Nina Olsson

KYLE BOOKS

Published in 2017 by Kyle Books
www.kylebooks.com

Distributed by National Book Network
4501 Forbes Blvd, Suite 200,
Lanham, MD 20706
Phone: (800) 462-6420
Fax: (800) 338-4550
customercare@nbnbooks.com

First published in Great Britain in 2017 by
Kyle Books, an imprint of Kyle Cathie Ltd.

10 9 8 7 6 5 4 3 2 1

ISBN 978-1-909487-69-7

Text © 2017 Nina Olsson
Design © 2017 Kyle Books
Photography © 2017 Nina Olsson

Nina Olsson is hereby identified as the author of this work in accordance with
Section 77 of the Copyright, Designs and Patents Act 1988.

All rights reserved. No reproduction, copy, or transmission of this publication may
be made without written permission. No paragraph of this publication may be
reproduced, copied, or transmitted save with written permission or in accordance
with the provisions of the Copyright Act 1956 (as amended). Any person who
does any unauthorized act in relation to this publication may be liable to criminal
prosecution and civil claims for damages.

Photographer, stylist and designer: Nina Olsson
Project Editor: Sophie Allen
Copy Editor: Stephanie Evans
Editorial Assistant: Hannah Coughlin
Production: Nic Jones, Gemma John, and Lisa Pinnell

Library of Congress Control Number: 2017938382

Color reproduction by ALTA, London.
Printed and bound in China by 1010 International Printing Ltd.

CONTENTS

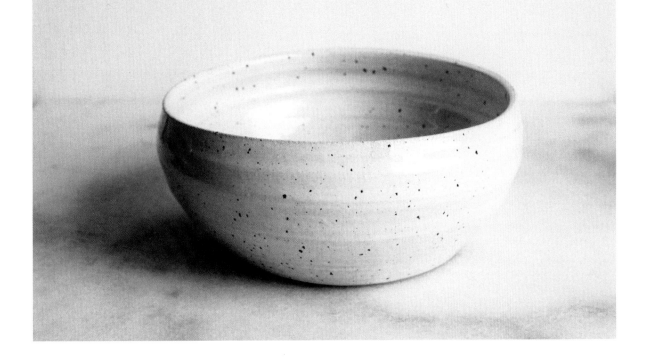

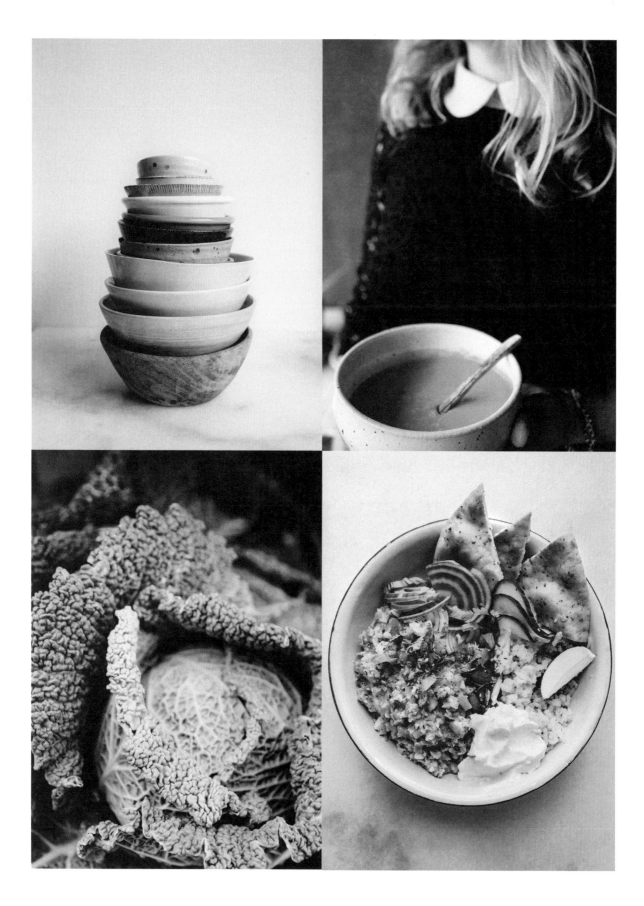

Bringing back the bowl

This cookbook is full of easy, delectable bowl meals. It's for everyone who likes to eat healthy, delicious, and comforting food with flavors from around the world. I've gathered some of my favorite vegetarian bowl-food recipes, covering everything from breakfast and dinner to small gatherings, to create casual, one-course dishes that layer texture and flavor.

Growing up in the seventies, I was lucky enough to be born in a time when home cooking was the norm and microwave ovens were a thing of sci-fi novels. I remember, with a mixture of horror and nostalgia, my family's transition during the eighties from comforting bakes and slow-cooked stews to defrosted microwave dinners. My parents were always busy, so quick solutions to feed the family were welcome. By the time I moved into my first home I felt an intuitive need to go in the opposite direction—by baking my own bread and eating mostly whole grains and whole foods. I prefer to make my own food from scratch as often as possible.

The way we are eating is rapidly changing. We are becoming more conscious about what we eat and interest in food over the past decade has risen to the same heights as popular music and fashion. Social media platforms like Instagram mirror our tastes and desires, creating snowball effects of likes and followers that carve out current trends in food culture.

That's where the story of this book begins. When my editor at Kyle Books approached me with the idea of making a cookbook about bowl food, it immediately appealed to me, as it illustrates the way I (and many others) like to eat today.

The bowl is not only a beautiful vessel, but a symbol that resonates with healthy and mindful eating, encompassing many of the good ideas about food that are popular now. One of the great advantages of bowl eating is that it's truly comforting. Perhaps it connects us with our ancient past. Evidence of the human tradition of eating from bowls can be found from archaeological digs all over the world. Our ancestors enjoyed their meals in bowls of wood, coconut shell, terracotta, glass, and porcelain, just as we do today.

In today's complex world, many of us look for ways to connect back to our roots by simplifying our lifestyle. We've learned the unpleasant truth about processed food—it is less nutritious and the industrialization of food production has given us overly sugary and additive-rich foods that tire our digestive system or, even worse, make us ill. We feel uncomfortable buying and eating eggs and dairy from herds reared with growth hormones and manufactured feeds. Large-scale meat production leaves much to be desired, as do the conditions for animals that are often appalling, to say the least. There's a growing number of people reclaiming the way we eat, who want to eat consciously, ethically, and healthfully. This book aims to inspire good, wholesome eating for all kinds of tastes.

Bowl eating is more often connected with a whole-food approach—a conscious decision to embrace the nutritional qualities of natural, raw ingredients—which has less in common with plated haute cuisine and refined ingredients. It's really an everyday kind of eating. Bowl food is generally fresh and healthy, with influences from authentic world kitchens. Still, bowl food is ultra-modern in our age! The ease of making bowl food from any leftover grains, fresh vegetables, and filling protein makes it a practical choice. Minimal fuss over food prepping and cooking go hand-in-hand with bowl eating; we're bringing back the bowl as our number-one everyday serving vessel because it is serving our purpose.

Making good choices

BALANCE

Choosing healthy can be confusing, with the jungle of voices and advice on offer. My definition of eating well is really simple: eat with variety and in moderation—it's the best health insurance you can invest in. I'm a big fan of light food, and it's clear that in the industrialized world people are generally over-saturated with calories, which is causing an alarming rise in obesity, diabetes, and heart disease. Both under- and overeating saps our energy. Naturally, we need to eat more when we are physically active and less when we are not. A healthy weight is a long-term project—quick fixes and diets are often working against us. Having a health-conscious attitude about eating is good, but be wary of developing fixations and unhealthy relationships with food—it should be enjoyed without guilt. It's better to be relaxed about it and have the occasional doughnut if you want to, as long as you maintain a healthy balance.

A PLANT-BASED DIET

A vegetarian diet can seem extreme to some, but it's a natural and nourishing way to eat. Many cultures around the world have a tradition of vegetarianism dating back thousands of years. Science and health authorities are pretty much in agreement that a plant-based diet is the most vital way to eat. Today, more and more people are choosing a vegan lifestyle. As long as you eat with variety and make sure you're getting the nutrients you need, you're eating well. Plant-based food is climate-smart too, using less energy and water than it takes to produce meat and fish.

THE NATURAL CHOICE

I choose to buy organic food when possible, especially for soy products that are most likely genetically modified if they're not organic. Genetically modified (GM) foods are possibly harmless for our health, and our history of eating this kind of food is relatively short, so it's a gamble to eat lots of it, unless you want to be an unofficial scientific experiment. Another issue with GM foods is that these crops are threatening the natural diversity of original seeds. Farmers worldwide have reacted with despair at the dependency on global seed manufacturers who restrict the varieties of plants grown for food to a few favored for their reliability, not quality. Genetically modified foods are not the standard everywhere, of course, and several countries have placed restrictions on GM crops to protect the environment. Supporting small-scale, organic farming is a good thing.

THE ECONOMY OF FOOD

I'd like to think that I make a positive contribution to the world when I buy food, so I choose Fairtrade where possible. It's a widely supported idea that poverty in developing countries can be overcome by supporting small-scale farming and businesses. The more Fairtrade we buy, the more we can help people to move from poverty to sustainability and independence. Of course not everyone is able to make the most ethical, environmental, and health-conscious choices when buying food. Health food, especially organic products, can have a hefty price tag. In most cases, though, there are good budget options that are just a little less hip. And the most essential healthy foods are cheap—kale, spinach, whole grains, beans, and lentils, for example. Careful food planning and prepping can save you money and reduce waste. Cooking from scratch is also great for keeping within a tight budget.

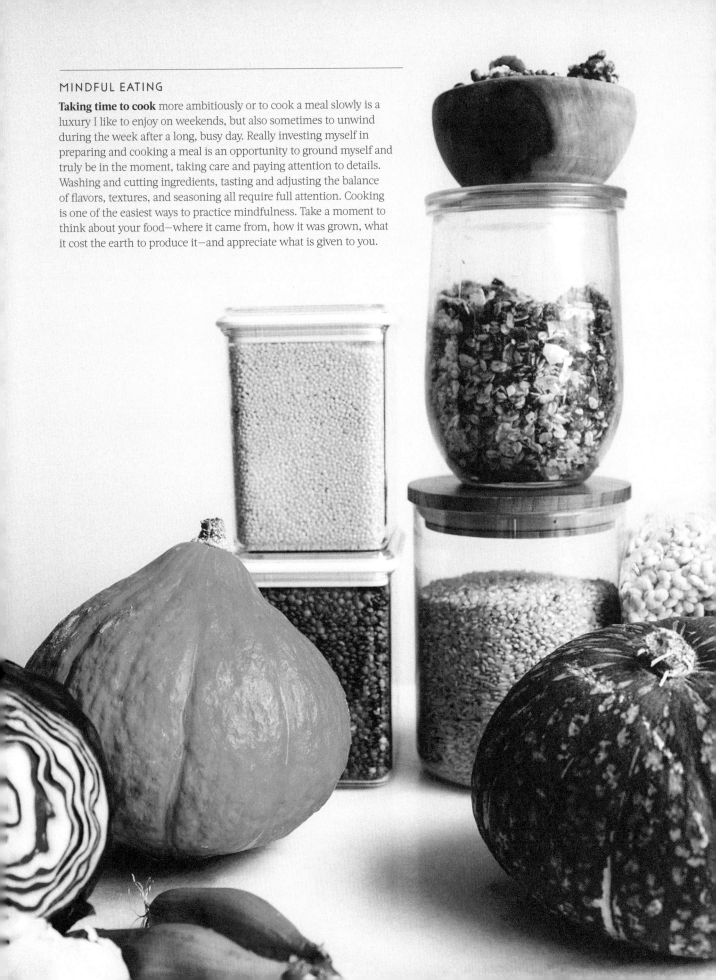

MINDFUL EATING

Taking time to cook more ambitiously or to cook a meal slowly is a luxury I like to enjoy on weekends, but also sometimes to unwind during the week after a long, busy day. Really investing myself in preparing and cooking a meal is an opportunity to ground myself and truly be in the moment, taking care and paying attention to details. Washing and cutting ingredients, tasting and adjusting the balance of flavors, textures, and seasoning all require full attention. Cooking is one of the easiest ways to practice mindfulness. Take a moment to think about your food—where it came from, how it was grown, what it cost the earth to produce it—and appreciate what is given to you.

Bowl food essentials

FOOD PREPPING

A little bit of planning and smart cooking saves a lot of time. Cook larger batches of grains, beans, and lentils and store them in the fridge to use later in the week.

For the dedicated prepper, choose a weeknight or weekend afternoon to prepare for the coming week: make pickles and salad dressings, hummus or other spreads, and cook large batches of your favorite grains and legumes. I also like to roast one or two trays of vegetables to use in salads, or blend into soups or dipping sauces. I keep grilled vegetables in jars with a little olive oil, herbs, and/or garlic. Whenever you have plenty of something—freeze it!

THE BASIC PANTRY

A base of beans, lentils, and whole grains is useful to have readily at home. They're great fillers and will give you plenty of good nutrition. Complement with nuts and seeds, vegetables, and fruit. These basic ingredients can be greatly varied with cooking techniques and some interesting add-ons.

COMPOSING A BOWL

A great bowl has a variety of textures. The key lies in balancing contrasts. Mix raw and cooked with roasted, toasted, and puréed elements. Topping salads with toasted nuts adds a delicious crunch and good fats. Avocado makes a perfect creamy addition. I like to match savory with refreshing, cooling ingredients such as mint, ginger, apple, or cucumber. Another way to enhance savory flavors is to add sweetness. Use a little agave syrup or honey in your sauces or dressings, or add a fruit or berries to a savory dish. Keep a neutral base of grains and fresh greens next to more interesting elements, such as spiced tempeh or toasted chickpeas. A little bit of tartness gives a great finish to most dishes. I alternate citrus fruits with vinegars or other components such as yogurt or pickles.

PLANT-BASED PROTEIN

Where meat eaters would add chicken, fish, or meat, vegetarians add plant protein. Popular choices are tofu and tempeh, made of soy beans. Tempeh is firmer and made from fermented beans, making it a healthier choice. Beans and lentils rate high on the satisfaction scale and make a great base in salads, stews, and soups. Another favorite of mine is seitan, a by-product of yeast-making. Seitan is sold in brine and sometimes flavored with soy or garlic. It comes in chunks and resembles meat more than tofu.

Seeds, seaweed, and nutritional yeast are also high in protein and add interest to neutral ingredients. Find tofu, tempeh, nutritional yeast, and seitan in health-food shops.

FLAVORING INGREDIENTS

At the heart of my savory dishes are umami-enriching ingredients, such as Japanese soy or tamari sauce, garlic and onions, mushrooms, seaweed, and nutritional yeast. I use a fair amount of citrus, such as lime, lemon, and orange, to add fresh notes, especially in Asian- and Middle Eastern-influenced dishes. I'm also nuts about nuts! Toast and sprinkle them over food, or grind into pastes such as tahini. Tahini, made from ground sesame seeds, is good in dressings, stews, and soups—it adds a full and complex flavor. Some other favorites are almonds and peanuts. Coconut is also in almost constant use in my kitchen, whether it's in the form of oil, milk, flakes, or desiccated flesh. I often combine the latter with peanuts for Indonesian-influenced cooking.

Herbs and spices add magic to food and I use both fresh and dried ones generously, including cumin, tarragon, cinnamon, oregano, thyme, basil, dill, and coriander. For spiciness, I use a variety of chile peppers, both fresh, dried, or in prepared sauces. It's best to pick the chile that fits with your inspiration—jalapeños for Mexican, shichimi togarishi for Japanese, and so on—but they can mostly be interchanged with perfect results.

How to use this book:

Plant-based and gluten-free alternatives are marked:
VE ✓ GF ✓

By suggesting vegan substitutes (VE) where there's dairy or eggs in the recipe you can opt to make your bowl fully plant-based. I've also added gluten-free options (GF) on almost all recipes.

I've kept down the salt dosage and generally suggest that you carefully season to taste, keeping salt on the table for guests who want to add more.

For sweetening, I use mostly coconut sugar and agave syrup. You can easily use brown or white sugar, honey, or other syrup instead as your sweetener. In general, all ingredients can be substituted for similar foods.

Although this book is vegetarian, many of the recipes will work for a flexitarian household by adjusting the ingredients to include fish and meat, but hopefully this book will inspire you to have fun with plant-based eating!

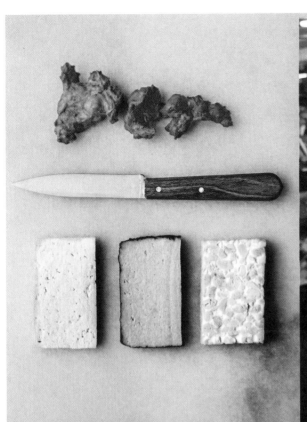
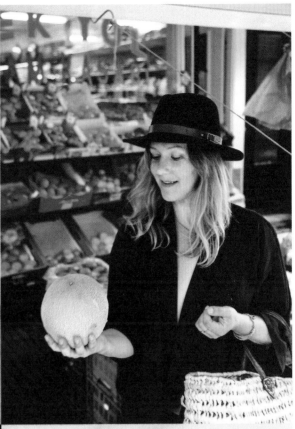
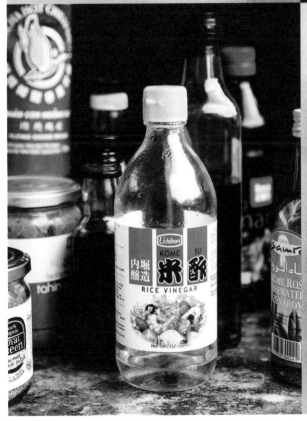
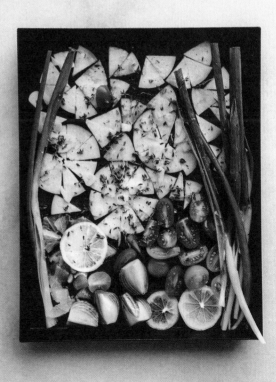

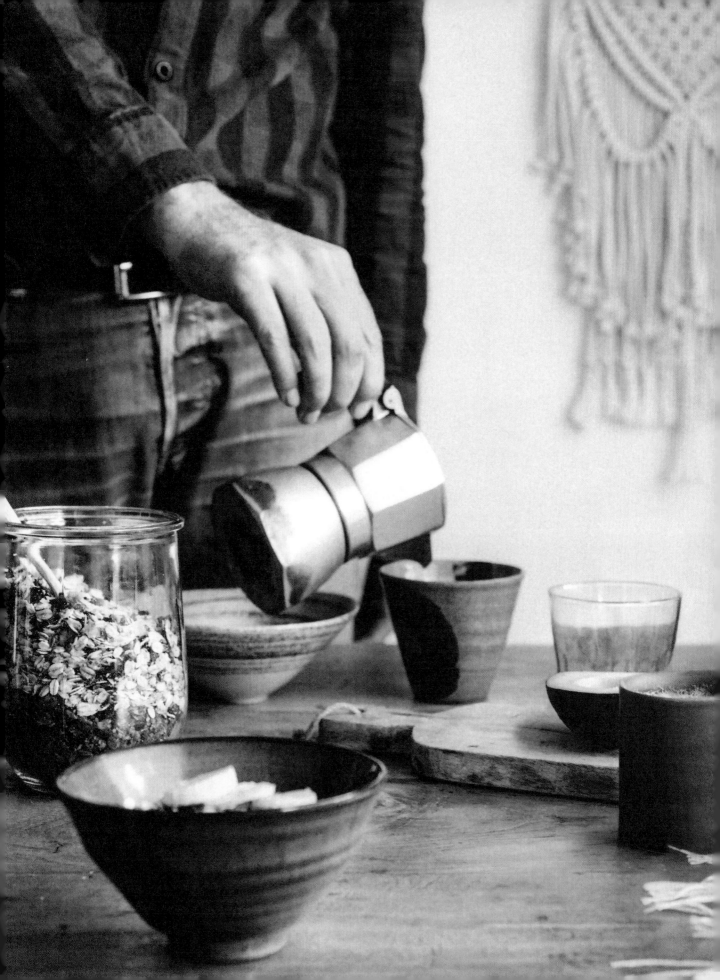

GOOD MORNING, SUNSHINE

Mornings are often the most challenging time to make good food choices. It's almost too easy to cut corners with sugary cereals and lattes "on the go." Since I started paying close attention to the relationship between my meals and my energy levels, I've learned how to avoid midday fatigue by starting the day with a wholesome breakfast. When time is in short supply, smoothies or overnight oats are what you need for sustainable energy. On weekends and holidays, a good breakfast can turn into a long brunch, and this can be the perfect time to enjoy a bowl of shakshuka or homemade granola with a cup of coffee.

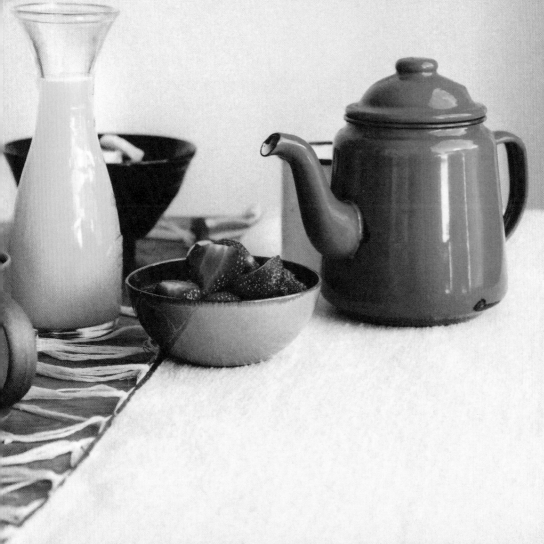

Kasha with Rhubarb and Peanut Butter

BUCKWHEAT PORRIDGE WITH RHUBARB AND PEAR COMPOTE

Buckwheat has a lot going for it. It's gluten-free, adapts to both savory and sweet dishes, and is full of good nutrition. It's actually not a grain but a seed and has a nutty, slightly bitter flavor when cooked. Kasha—buckwheat porridge—is made by toasting the buckwheat before simmering, which intensifies its nutty flavor. The delicious rhubarb and pear compote adds tangy sweetness and the spoonful of peanut butter a creamy, savory finish.

For the rhubarb compote, add the ingredients to a small saucepan and bring to a boil. Simmer for 5 minutes and remove from heat. Set aside to cool.

For the porridge, heat a small saucepan and melt the coconut oil. Add the buckwheat and stir until golden. Add the milk and a pinch of salt. Simmer slowly for 15 minutes or until the milk is absorbed. Remove from the heat and stir the syrup and vanilla extract into the porridge. Serve with rhubarb compote, a splash of cold milk, and a spoonful of peanut butter.

VE ✓ GF ✓

SERVES 4

RHUBARB AND PEAR COMPOTE
$\frac{1}{2}$ lb. rhubarb (about 3 stalks), trimmed and chopped
2 pears, halved, peeled, and cored
juice of 1 orange
1 teaspoon freshly grated ginger
$\frac{1}{4}$ cup coconut sugar or brown sugar

PORRIDGE
1 teaspoon coconut oil
$\frac{3}{4}$ cup buckwheat, soaked overnight and drained
$1\frac{1}{4}$ cups almond milk
2 tablespoons maple or agave syrup
few drops of vanilla extract
salt

TO SERVE
almond milk or milk of your choice
1 tablespoon natural peanut butter

GOODNESS GRAINESS! *Eating whole grains daily is a sure way of getting many of the important nutrients we need, keeping our digestive system healthy, and our weight in check. Too many people miss out on the benefits of grains by choosing refined products instead of the whole grain. Eating whole grains decreases the chances of developing serious diseases, such as diabetes and heart problems.*

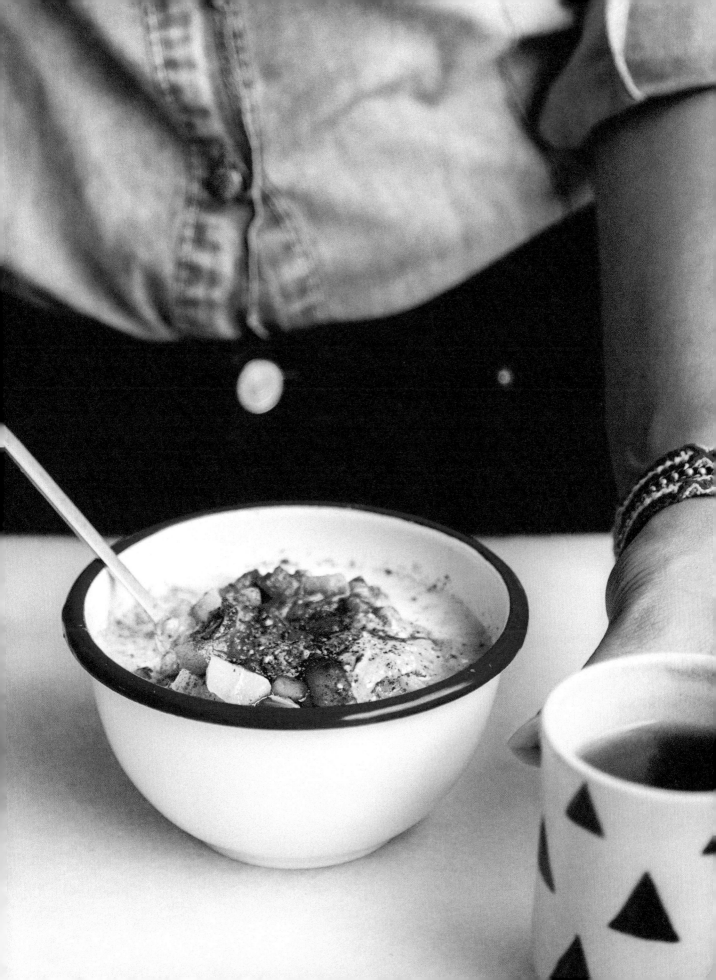

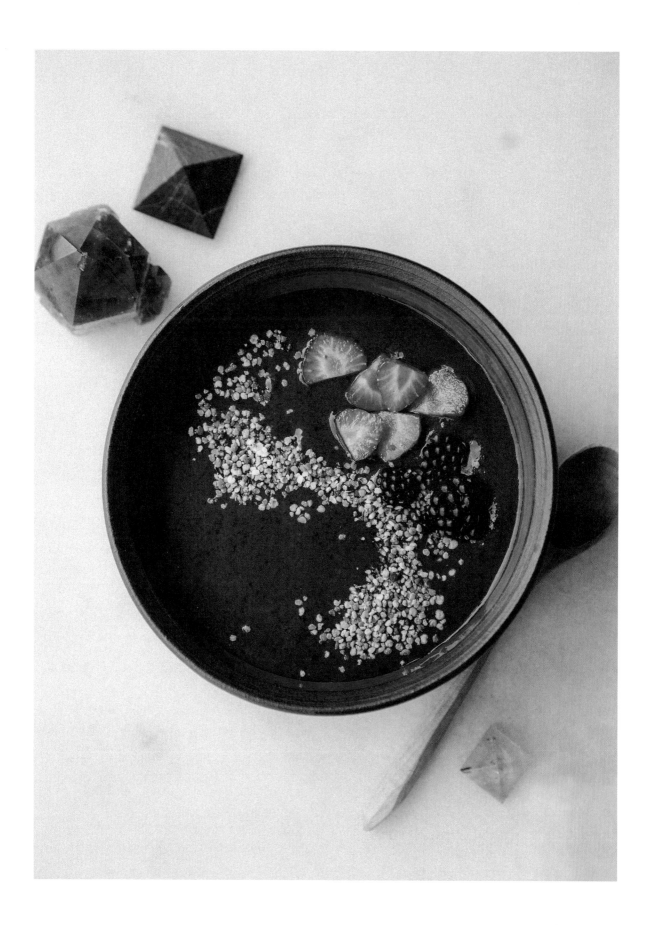

Blueberry Açaí Bowl

BLUEBERRY-AÇAÍ SMOOTHIE BOWL WITH BEE POLLEN AND BERRIES

What's not to love about smoothies? They're quick, delicious, and healthy. My freezer is always stocked with frozen berries, bananas, and other fruit. All they need to become a quick breakfast is blending with coconut water or nut milk.

Making smoothies offers a great opportunity to sneak superfoods such as wheatgrass, raw cacao, and açaí into your diet, and here it's the açaí berry that gives this smoothie bowl its beautiful red and purple color. This Brazilian gem has been widely praised for its health benefits, but it's the bittersweet flavor that's the real winner.

Topping a smoothie bowl is all about adding something pretty and healthy. I like to give this a galactic look with a sprinkle of bee pollen.

Blend the bowl ingredients until smooth and creamy. Pour into a bowl and top with colorful fruit and superfoods.

Tip! You can buy açaí purée packets or powder in health food stores or online. If you wish, substitute other berries for açaí.

VE *Choose agave syrup and omit bee pollen.*
GF ✓

SERVES 1
1 cup açaí purée
½ cup blueberries
⅔ cup coconut water
1 ripe banana, peeled
1 avocado, pitted and peeled
2 tablespoons almond butter
1 teaspoon agave syrup or honey
few drops of vanilla extract

SUGGESTIONS FOR TOPPINGS
chunks of raw fruit—passion fruit, dragon fruit, pineapple, kiwi, kumquats, strawberries, and other berries are all good
coconut flakes
nuts and seeds, such as hemp
bee pollen
cacao nibs

Stockholm Scramble

TOFU SCRAMBLE WITH DILL, CHIVES, GARLIC, AND RYE CRISPBREAD

I often alternate scrambled eggs with tofu scramble. Tofu is a blank canvas when it comes to flavor and this recipe is made using classic Scandinavian tastes of pine nuts, red onion, and fresh dill, served with rustic rye crispbread (knäckebröd). These are the flavors I love to share with friends and family in Stockholm. Here the tofu takes extra zest and character from chives and garlic. The addition of wholesome spinach and avocado means this breakfast will load you with good energy for the day.

Blend the pine nuts, nutritional yeast (if using), and salt to a crumble in a food processor or with a mortar and pestle. Set aside. Press the tofu between two plates with paper towels under the tofu to soak up excess liquid, then crumble it finely with your hands or a fork. Heat a skillet over medium-high heat. Add the oil and stir-fry the onion until translucent. Add the crumbled tofu and season with salt and pepper.

Add the garlic and herbs and stir for 2 to 3 minutes. Add the spinach and remove from the heat when it's just wilted. Season to taste. Divide the tofu scramble between four serving bowls. Top with avocado slices and the pine nut sprinkle. Serve with crispbread spread with cream cheese and radishes.

Tip! For a seaweed twist, use Japanese rice seasoning (furikake) instead of the pine nut sprinkle.

VE *Use vegan cream cheese instead of regular cream cheese.*

GF *Serve with gluten-free crackers instead of crispbread.*

SERVES 4

PINE NUT SPRINKLE
½ cup pine nuts, crushed
2 tablespoons nutritional yeast (optional)
½ teaspoon salt

TOFU SCRAMBLE
14 oz. firm tofu
2 tablespoons vegetable oil
1 red onion, finely chopped
2 garlic cloves, finely chopped to a paste
big bunch of fresh chives, chopped
handful of fresh dill, chopped
5–6 oz. spinach or other leafy greens, washed and finely chopped
2 avocados, pitted, peeled, and thinly sliced
salt and pepper

TO SERVE
slices of crispbread or dark rye bread
cream cheese (or vegan cream cheese)
bunch of radishes, halved

THIS IS TOFU: *Tofu is made from curdled soy milk and is a good protein source for vegans and vegetarians. It's also an exceptional plant food as it contains all eight of the essential amino acids that humans need. It has been eaten in Asia for centuries and is truly versatile—good in both savory and sweet dishes. Buy your tofu from natural health food stores or look for packaging marked certified GMO-free to get the good stuff.*

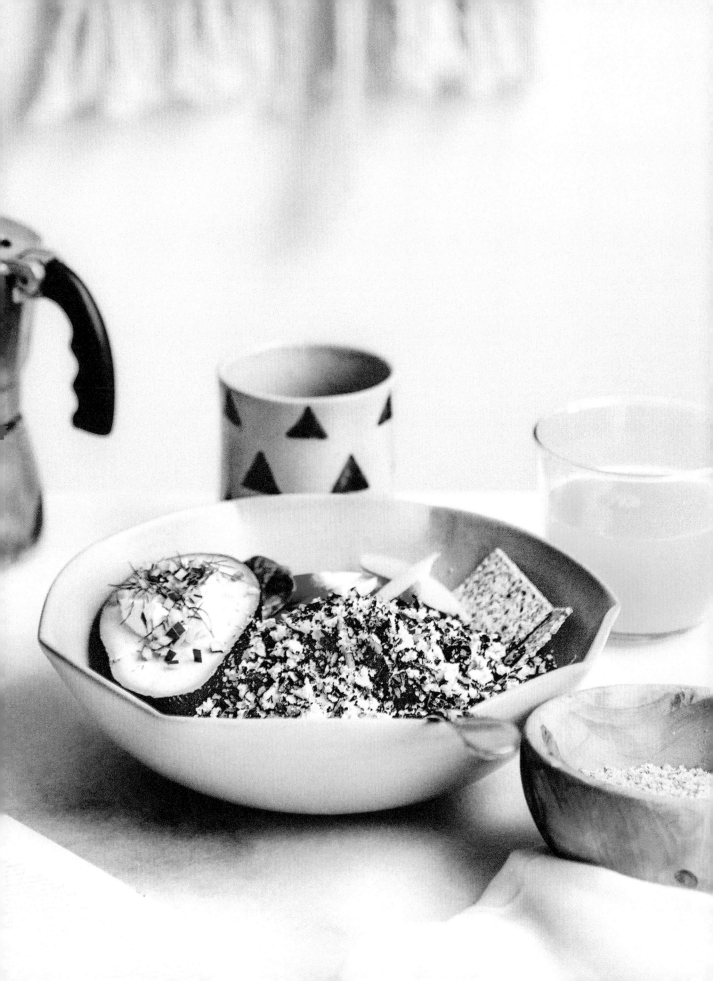

The Green Queen

POACHED EGG AND SMASHED AVOCADO TOAST WITH MISO AND CARROT DRESSING

This recipe is inspired by The Green Queen café in Stockholm, where they serve a mean avocado smash and poached egg breakfast with delicious sauce. The creamy avocado and soft yolk are balanced by crunchy toast, radishes, and nuts. To spice it all up, drizzle with fermented miso and carrot dressing or your favorite hot sauce!

Poaching eggs can be intimidating until you've learned the technique, but it's very easy. Bring a saucepan of water to a simmer, whip up a good swirl in the water, and let your raw egg gently float into the stream. After a few minutes you will have a silky smooth warm egg.

Crush the bigger nuts and mix with the smaller nuts and seeds in a bowl. Sprinkle in salt and red pepper flakes to taste.

Whisk the ingredients for the miso and carrot dressing until smooth. Arrange the radishes and tomatoes in a bowl with the green leaves. Drizzle 1 tablespoon lemon juice over the avocado and mash with a fork. Lightly season with salt and pepper and add to the bowl.

Fill a small saucepan with water and bring to a simmer over medium-high heat. Gently crack the egg into a cup. Create a swirl in the simmering water with a whisk and carefully slip the egg into the swirl in one smooth movement. Let the egg firm up for 4 minutes then gently remove it from the water with a slotted spoon and drain on paper towels. Add the poached egg to the bowl. Season to taste. Top with the salted, red pepper-nut sprinkle and a drizzle of miso and carrot dressing. Serve with sourdough toast.

Tip! The dressing can be prepared in advance as it keeps in the fridge for days. This recipe makes enough to store and use again in the coming days.

VE *Omit the egg or substitute tofu scramble.*
GF *Use gluten-free bread.*

SERVES 1

handful of mixed seeds and toasted nuts (hemp seeds, pine nuts, almonds, walnuts, etc.)
red pepper flakes
3–4 radishes, trimmed and sliced
4–5 cherry tomatoes, halved
handful of vibrant green leaves (I used spinach)
1 avocado, pitted and peeled
juice of $\frac{1}{2}$ lemon
1 free-range egg
salt and pepper

MISO AND CARROT DRESSING
(makes about 1 cup)
$\frac{1}{4}$ cup white or yellow miso paste
$\frac{1}{4}$ cup rice vinegar
$2\frac{1}{2}$ tablespoons extra-virgin olive oil
1 carrot, grated
1 teaspoon freshly grated ginger
$\frac{1}{2}$ teaspoon Sriracha or other hot sauce (optional)
2 tablespoons toasted sesame oil
$2\frac{1}{2}$ tablespoons agave syrup

TO SERVE
1 slice sourdough toast

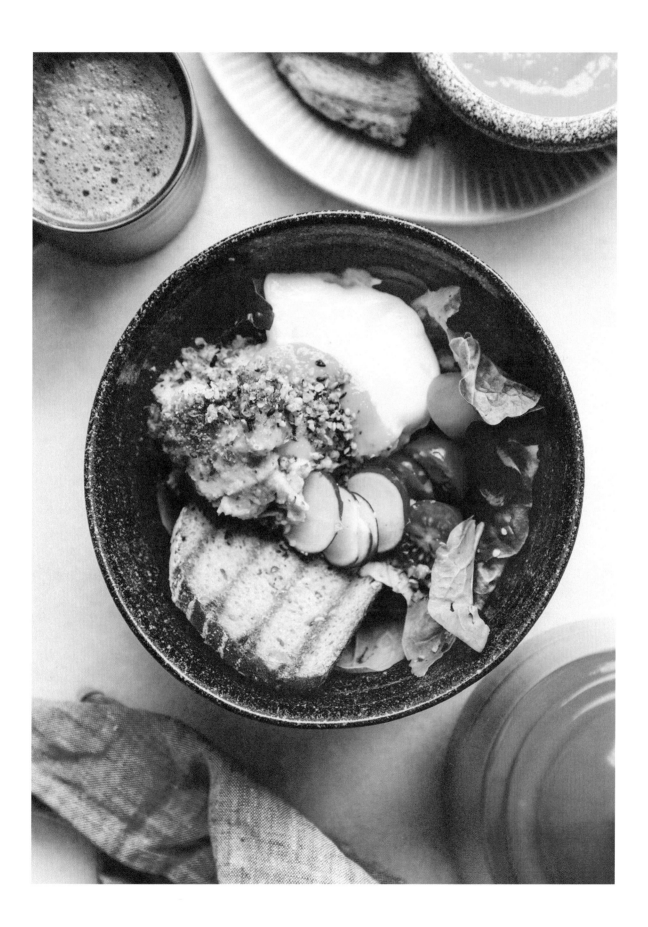

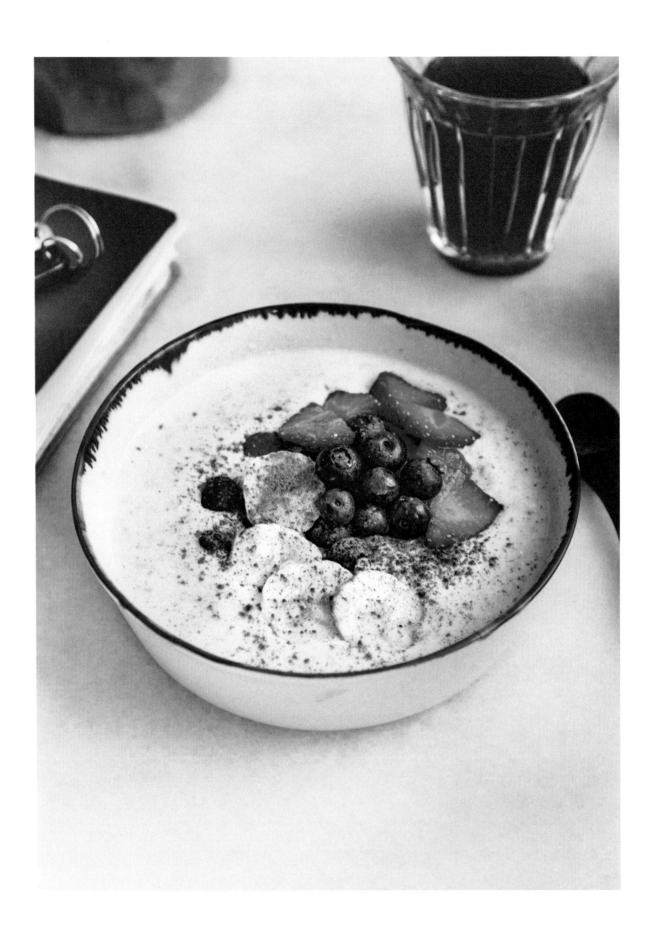

Overnight Oats

CREAMY NO-COOK, RAW OAT PORRIDGE

My childhood breakfast of choice was cinnamon-scented oatmeal. I soon learned how to cook it myself and discovered that the longer the oats cooked, the tastier the result. I'm still a big fan of oatmeal for breakfast and this raw version in particular. Soaking the oats overnight slowly turns them into a bowl of silky creaminess and helps to break down the phytic acid—a natural defense component in all plants that is harmful to humans in large doses—more effectively than regular cooking does.

This breakfast is incredibly easy and fuss-free to make! All you need to do is mix oats and liquid in a bowl and leave overnight. The next morning you can just grab a spoon and eat it immediately—no time spent stirring, no pots to clean. The basic recipe can be made with a variation of stir-ins and toppings.

Mix the oats and chia seeds, if using, with the juice, milk, and yogurt in a bowl and cover. Place in the fridge overnight. In the morning, stir in maple syrup and a pinch of salt, then mix with a spoon. Add your choice of stir-ins and toppings and it's ready to eat.

VE *Use a plant-based yogurt like soygurt or coconut yogurt.*
GF *Check that your oats are certified free from gluten contamination.*

MAKES 1 BOWL

1 cup ground (Scottish style) oats
1 tablespoon chia seeds (optional)
²⁄₃ cup natural apple juice (or other juice)
¼ cup nut or oat milk
¼ cup Greek yogurt

STIR-INS AND TOPPINGS

1 teaspoon maple syrup or honey
pinch of salt
few drops of vanilla extract
1 heaping spoon blueberries, smashed, 1–2 strawberries, or chunks of other fresh fruit or berries
cinnamon
1–2 tablespoons nut butter (try peanut butter)
nuts and seeds
raw cacao nibs

Rose and Pistachio Granola

ROSE-SCENTED GRANOLA WITH HINTS OF BAKLAVA

I was thinking of Turkish baklava—a popular Middle Eastern pastry layered with pistachios and honey—when I came up with this recipe. Rose and pistachio make a famous flavor combination and one that is frequently used in Iranian cooking; adding rose to the baklava flavor gives this granola an extra romantic element and it's like eating a crumbled cookie or a healthy dessert for breakfast. Serve it with yogurt, pomegranate seeds, or fresh berries and rose petals.

Preheat the oven to 350°F and line a baking sheet with parchment. Mix the vanilla extract with the oil, honey, and tahini. Spread the oats, almonds, pistachios, coconut flakes, sesame seeds, and rose petals onto the baking sheet. Drizzle the oil and honey mixture over the dry ingredients, making sure the oats and nuts are well coated. Dust lightly with the cardamom and cinnamon, toss lightly. Spread evenly and sprinkle with a small bit of salt. Bake for 15 to 20 minutes, checking every few minutes to make sure it doesn't burn.

Cool and store in a large jar with a tight-fitting lid. Serve with Greek yogurt or labneh, topped with rose petals and pomegranate seeds, berries, or a spoonful of jam.

VE *Use vegan yogurt.*

GF *Check that your oats are certified free from gluten contamination.*

MAKES A BIG JAR
(about 2 pounds)

$1/4$ teaspoon vanilla extract
$1/3$ cup olive oil
$1/4$ cup clear honey or agave syrup
1 teaspoon tahini
$2 1/4$ cups rolled oats
$3/4$ cup almonds, sliced
1 cup pistachios, crushed
$3 1/4$ cup coconut flakes
$1/4$ cup sesame seeds
edible rose petals, dry or fresh
$1/2$ tablespoon ground cardamom
$1/2$ teaspoon ground cinnamon
salt

TO SERVE
Greek yogurt or labneh
rose petals
pomegranate seeds, berries, or jam

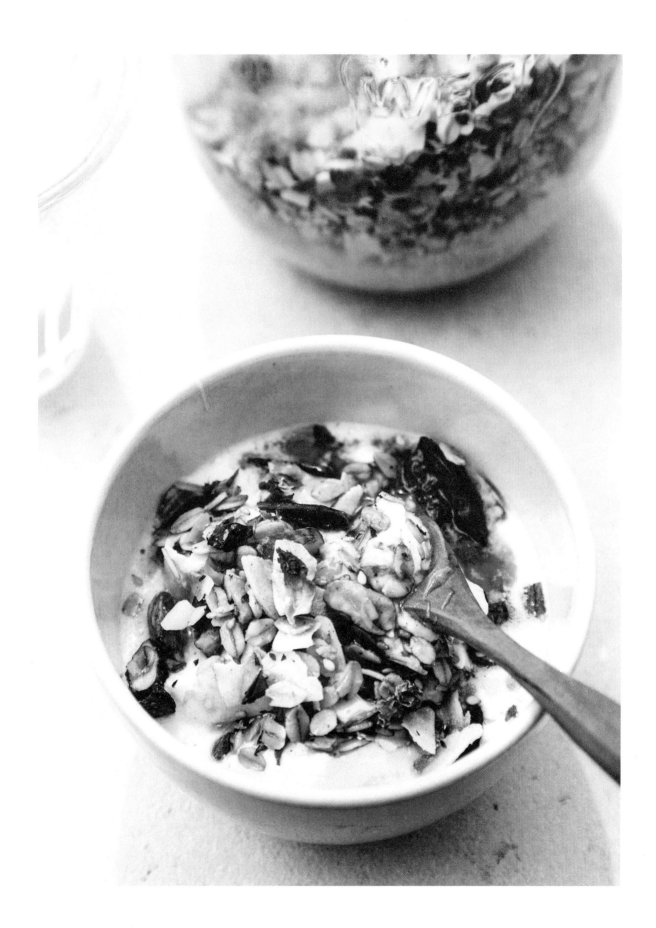

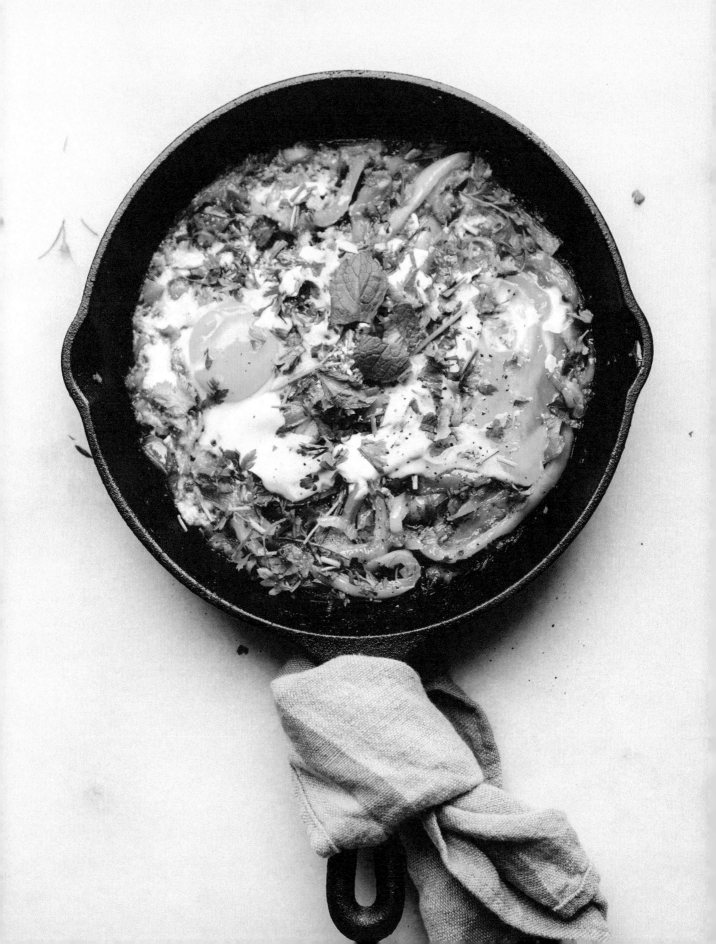

Golden Shakshuka

ONIONS, PEPPERS, AND EGGS IN CUMIN AND TURMERIC SAUCE

The vibrant flavors of shakshuka have spread its popularity far beyond the Middle East, and it is a real success in our house on weekend mornings.

Slowly cooking cumin, onion, tomatoes, and peppers makes an irresistible base for the poached eggs in this one-pan dish. The time invested in letting the ingredients slowly break apart is rewarded with deep, sweet, pan-roasted flavor. This recipe is a twist on the classic red shakshuka—using turmeric, yellow pepper, and yellow tomatoes makes a bright sunshine-yellow breakfast bowl. Scoop up the shakshuka with bread and serve with a cool yogurt sauce and fresh herbs.

Prepare the yogurt sauce by mixing the ingredients in a bowl, then set aside. Add a drizzle of olive oil to a skillet and place over medium-low heat. Stir-fry the onion until translucent, about 5 to 10 minutes.

Add the peppers, cumin, turmeric, thyme, ground coriander, and cayenne to the skillet. Stir to coat the onions and peppers with the spices. Add the cherry tomatoes and garlic-salt mixture and cook over low heat for 15 minutes, stirring frequently. If the sauce begins to dry out, add a little oil and water, but add sparingly as the shakshuka should not be watery.

Use the back of a spoon to make two shallow indentations in the surface of the shakshuka and crack an egg into each. Leave the shakshuka to slowly bake the eggs for 10 minutes, keeping the heat low. The result should be a dry sauce with the eggs just set. Remove from the heat.

Serve in bowls with the yogurt sauce drizzled over and top with fresh herbs and za'atar and enjoy with bread to scoop up the shakshuka sauce.

Tip! For a classic shakshuka, omit the turmeric and use red peppers and tomatoes.

VE *Omit the eggs. Instead, serve with avocado. Substitute vegan yogurt.*

GF *Use gluten-free bread or omit altogether.*

SERVES 2
olive oil
2 onions, thinly sliced
2 yellow bell peppers, thinly sliced
$\frac{1}{2}$ teaspoon ground cumin
$\frac{1}{2}$ teaspoon freshly grated turmeric
  or ground turmeric
$\frac{1}{2}$ teaspoon thyme (dried or fresh)
$\frac{1}{2}$ teaspoon ground coriander
pinch of cayenne pepper or
  $\frac{1}{2}$ teaspoon spicy harissa
2 cups yellow cherry tomatoes,
  chopped
2 garlic cloves, finely chopped to a
  paste with $\frac{1}{2}$ teaspoon salt
2 free-range eggs

YOGURT SAUCE
$\frac{1}{2}$ cup Greek yogurt
1 teaspoon honey
juice of $\frac{1}{2}$ lemon

TO SERVE
handful of fresh herbs (cilantro,
  mint, parsley), chopped
dusting of za'atar
fresh bread

Kale and Quinoa with Savory Granola

GARLICKY MUSHROOMS WITH WILTED GREENS, QUINOA, AND GRANOLA

With all the goodness in this bowl, making this breakfast is a pure act of self-love. Kale and quinoa, two powerhouses of nutrition, are on the A-list of healthy ingredients. And with good reason—they're both versatile to cook with and boost your well-being to the max. To make it even more interesting, add a savory granola for crunch and extra fiber.

To make the granola, heat a drizzle of olive oil in a skillet over medium-high heat and stir-fry the oats, pumpkin seeds, sesame seeds, almonds, and pine nuts until fragrant, about 4 to 5 minutes. Sprinkle with thyme, red pepper flakes, and salt, then remove from the heat.

Cook the quinoa according to the package instructions and drain. Remove any thick stalks from the greens and tear into pieces. Heat a drizzle of olive oil in a skillet over medium-high heat. Add the mushrooms and garlic, sauté until the mushrooms are brown, about 5 minutes. Add the scallions and greens and sprinkle with salt and red pepper flakes. Stir-fry until the greens are wilted, about 2 to 3 minutes. Remove from the heat, taste, and adjust the seasoning with salt and pepper.

Divide the quinoa, kale, and mushroom mixture into serving bowls. Top with some savory granola and add fresh cherry tomatoes and cottage cheese.

VE *Omit the cottage cheese.*
GF *Check your oats are certified free from gluten contamination.*

SERVES 4
¾ cup quinoa
3½ cups fresh green leaves, such as baby kale, baby spinach, and Swiss chard, washed and drained
olive oil
½ lb. brown mushrooms, brushed
2 garlic cloves, finely chopped to a paste
4–5 scallions, thinly sliced
pinch of red pepper flakes
salt and pepper

SAVORY GRANOLA
(makes about 2 cups)
drizzle of olive oil
1 cup rolled oats
½ cup pumpkin seeds
½ cup sesame seeds
½ cup almonds
½ cup pine nuts
1 tablespoon fresh or dried thyme
pinch of red pepper flakes
salt

TO SERVE
bunch of cherry tomatoes
½ cup cottage cheese

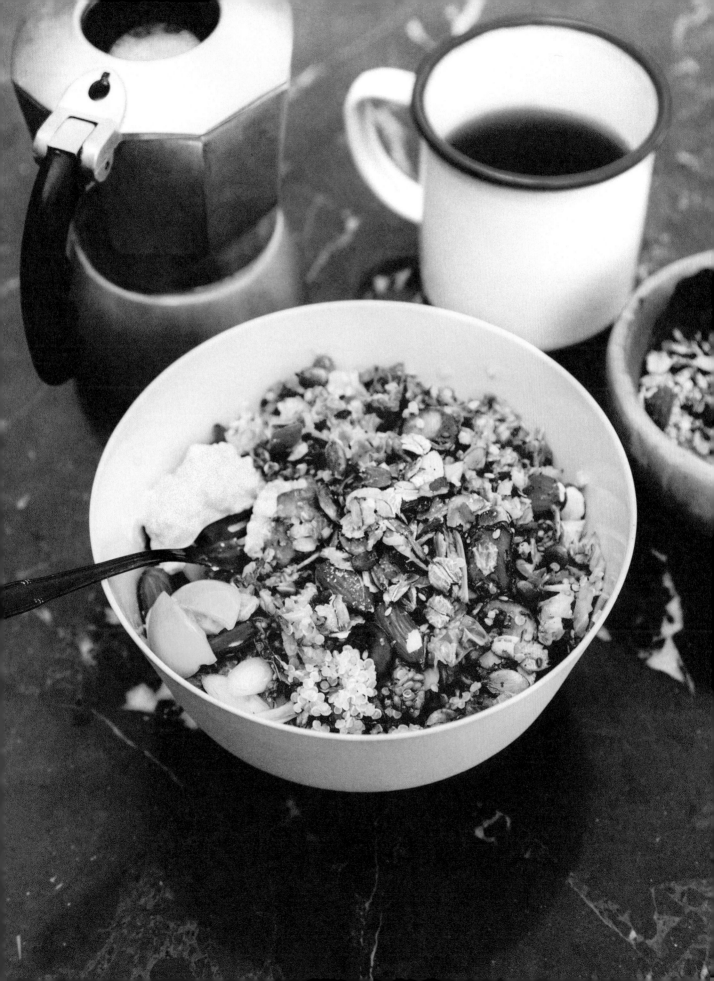

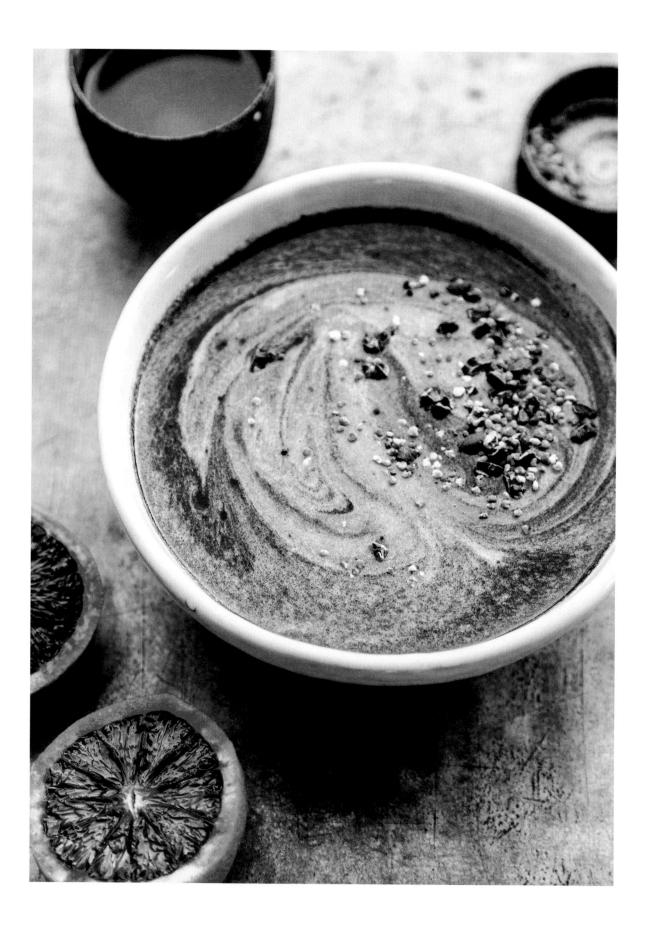

Cosmic Chlorella

VANILLA BANANA SMOOTHIE WITH CHLOROPHYLL-RICH ALGAE

This smoothie is a lifesaver when you're in a rush. Its healthfulness is enhanced by protein powder and superfood ingredients, including chlorella, a blue-green algae sold in health food shops that contains powerful nutritients of chlorophyll, amino acids, and B-complex vitamins. You can blend the chlorella with the base smoothie, or stir it in later, as I like to do, for a stunning cosmic swirl. For a contrasting kick, I also like to top with a squeeze of citrus juice—if blood oranges are in season, go for a sweet red citrus addition. For an extra-nourishing breakfast, top with bee pollen, puffed quinoa, cacao nibs, coconut flakes, or nuts and seeds.

This smoothie is really refreshing and light, but to make it more filling simply add healthy breakfast cereals, fruit, or berries.

Process the smoothie base in a blender and pour into a bowl. Swirl in the chlorella with a teaspoon then squeeze the juice of a blood orange in a swirl over the smoothie. Sprinkle with the toppings of your choice.

VE *Omit the bee pollen.*
GF ✓

MAKES 1 BOWL

BASE
1 scoop vanilla protein powder
1 cup nut, oat, or coconut milk
1 banana, peeled

STIR-INS
1 teaspoon chlorella
$\frac{1}{2}$ orange or blood orange

TOPPINGS (OPTIONAL)
bee pollen
puffed quinoa
cacao nibs
nuts and seeds, such as hemp

Green Beauty

SPIRULINA, AVOCADO, AND SPINACH SMOOTHIE

This creamy green power bowl will fuel you with one of the world's most nutritious foods, the blue-green algae spirulina. As a health supplement, I find spirulina has the strongest and quickest effect on both the health of my skin and my energy levels. However, it needs to be paired with other ingredients to take the edge off its strong flavor. Mixing it with banana and other fruits and vanilla does the trick. This smoothie has avocado and spinach for added green goodness, providing healthy oils, fiber, and vitamins.

I don't often sweeten my smoothies, but here I add agave syrup to balance the bitterness of the spirulina powder. It does depend on individual taste and habits, so adjust the sweetener to your preference.

Whizz the smoothie ingredients in a blender and pour into a bowl. Top with kiwi, strawberries, papaya, coconut, bee pollen, or any other superfood or fruit of your choice.

VE *Omit the bee pollen.*
GF ✓

MAKES 1 BOWL

1 avocado
1 tablespoon spirulina powder
1 small banana
handful of spinach
1 tablespoon almond butter
drizzle of olive oil
tiny pinch of salt
¼ teaspoon vanilla extract
half a mango or a quarter of a
   papaya, peeled, pit or seeds
   removed, and chopped
juice of 1 lemon
1 tablespoon agave syrup (optional)
⅔ cup nut or oat milk

TOPPINGS
kiwi, peeled and sliced
strawberries, halved
papaya, peeled and chopped
coconut pieces or sprinkles of
   desiccated or shredded coconut
bee pollen

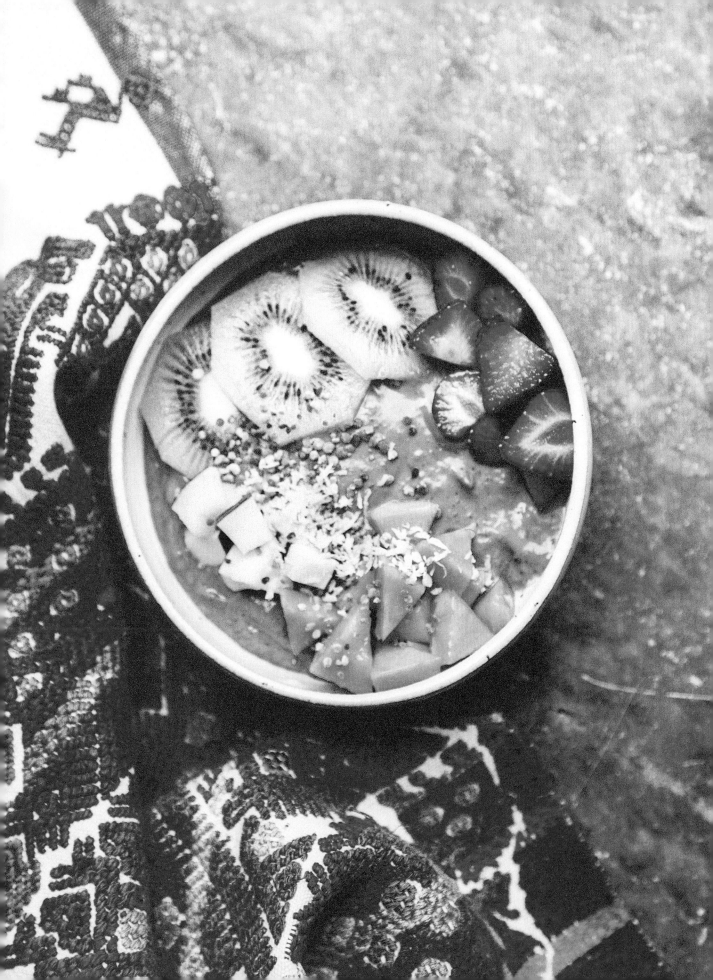

Lime and Strawberry Kisses

LIME STRAWBERRIES WITH CINNAMON AND VANILLA YOGURT

A breakfast of strawberries is one of life's sweetest pleasures and they are particularly delicious with a bit of tangy citrus. The Greek yogurt can be swapped out for other yogurts and vegan options such as soygurt or coconut yogurt. If you find organic yogurt with live bacteria culture, go for it, as it's great for your health.

SERVES 4

1½ cups strawberries, halved
juice of 1 lime
2 cups Greek yogurt or soygurt
2 tablespoons clear honey
pinch of salt
¼ teaspoon vanilla extract
½ teaspoon ground cinnamon

Fill a bowl with the strawberries and sprinkle with lime juice. In another bowl, stir the yogurt with the honey, salt, and vanilla. Divide the yogurt between serving bowls and top with the strawberries. Drizzle some additional honey over the strawberries and sprinkle with a little cinnamon. Garnish with extra lime wedges.

VE *Substitute vegan yogurt.*
GF ✓

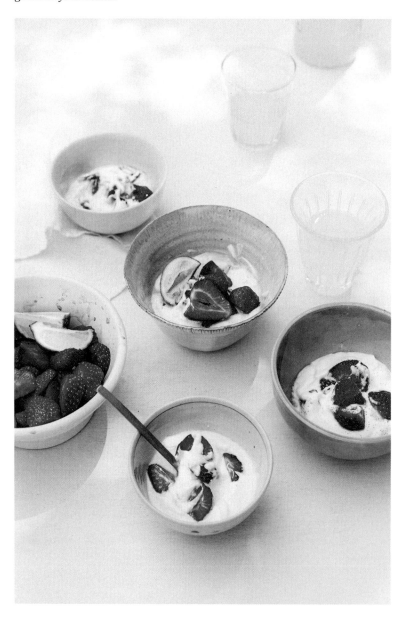

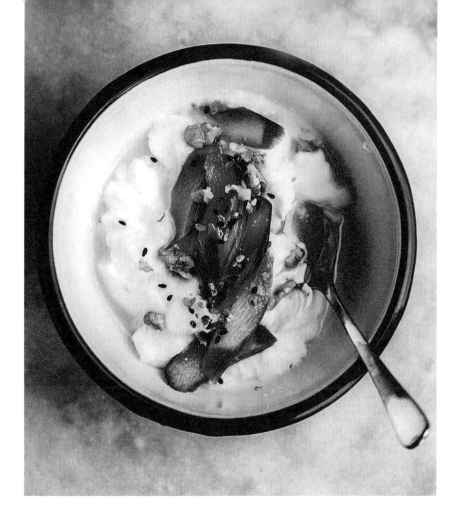

Rhubarb and Orange Yogurt

CARDAMOM AND VANILLA RHUBARB AND ORANGE YOGURT BOWL

Bright pink rhubarb and sweet orange make regular yogurt a lot more interesting for a light breakfast.

Place the rhubarb, orange juice, cardamom, agave syrup, and vanilla in a saucepan with enough water to just cover the rhubarb. Bring to a boil, then reduce the heat and simmer for 10 minutes. Remove from heat and add the orange blossom water before serving with yogurt. Top with nuts, seeds, and bee pollen.

VE *Substitute vegan yogurt.*
Omit the bee pollen.
GF ✓

SERVES 1
½ lb. rhubarb (2–3 stalks), chopped
juice of 1 orange
pinch of ground cardamom
¼ cup agave syrup
¼ teaspoon vanilla extract
few drops of orange blossom water
1 cup Greek yogurt

SUGGESTED TOPPINGS
1 tablespoon walnuts, crushed
sprinkle of black sesame seeds
sprinkle of bee pollen

Mexican Breakfast Bowl

QUINOA, TOFU, AND BLACK BEAN SCRAMBLE WITH LIME SAUCE

My love of tacos and Mexican food is undying, but I often skip the taco shells and make a salad bowl with my favorite Mexican flavors instead. This Mexican-inspired scramble is full of flavor and nutritious goodness.

Don't let the long list of ingredients discourage you from trying this recipe. It's really quick and easy, and you will probably have most of the ingredients, such as the spices, in your pantry already. The mouthwatering combination of lime, cilantro, mango, bean, and tofu scramble makes this a real super-bowl. I've added protein-rich quinoa—a nutritional powerhouse—to continue the Latin theme. The serving suggestions can be easily supplemented by your own favorite add-ons.

Cook the quinoa according to the package instructions. Drain and fluff with a fork, then set aside. Stir the Baja sauce ingredients into a smooth sauce. Refrigerate until ready to serve.

Mix the salsa ingredients and set aside.

To make the scramble, heat a skillet over medium-high heat and add a drizzle of canola oil. Stir-fry the tofu crumbles until golden, in batches if necessary, about 2 to 3 minutes. Transfer the tofu to a bowl.

Wipe out the pan and reheat over medium-high heat. Add another drizzle of oil and cook the red onion and garlic for 4 minutes on low heat until the onion is translucent. Add the black beans, tofu, quinoa, and corn and cook for 3 to 4 minutes over medium-low heat. Add the dry spices, then mix well and cook for 1 to 2 minutes more over low heat. Remove from heat and toss with the cilantro. Add salt and pepper to taste.

Divide the quinoa and bean scramble between four bowls. Serve with salsa, scallions, radishes, red cabbage, Baja sauce, hot sauce, grated cheese, and lime wedges. Add corn tortilla chips if you want that extra taco crunch.

VE *Substitute Vegenaise for mayonnaise and vegan crème fraîche for crème fraîche (see page 50). For grated cheese, use nutritional yeast or rawmesan (see page 55).*

GF *Use corn tortilla chips if you like to include tortillas.*

SERVES 4
1 cup quinoa

BAJA SAUCE
1/2 cup mayonnaise
1/2 cup crème fraîche
1 avocado, pitted, peeled, and chopped
pinch of salt
zest and juice of 1 lime

SALSA
1 mango, pitted, peeled, and diced
1 avocado, pitted, peeled, and diced
1 jalapeño pepper, seeded and finely chopped
juice of 1 lime
handful of cilantro and mint leaves, finely chopped

SCRAMBLE
canola oil
8 oz. smoked tofu, crumbled
1 red onion, diced
2 garlic cloves, finely chopped to a paste
14 1/2 oz. can black beans, rinsed and drained
8 oz. can corn kernels
1/2 teaspoon each of the following ground spices: cumin, oregano, black pepper
1 teaspoon paprika
1 teaspoon ground coriander
3/4 teaspoon salt
1/4 teaspoon cayenne pepper
handful of fresh cilantro, chopped
salt and pepper

TO SERVE
2 scallions, thinly sliced
4 radishes, thinly sliced
red cabbage, finely shredded
hot sauce (Sriracha or similar)
grated cheese or nutritional yeast
lime wedges
corn tortilla chips (optional)

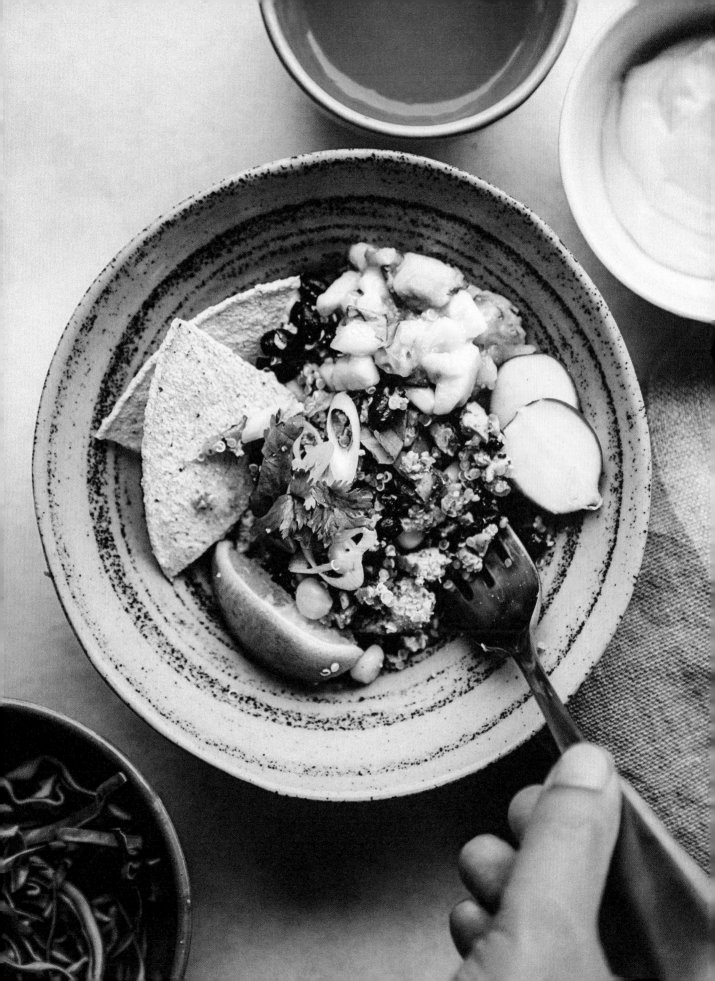

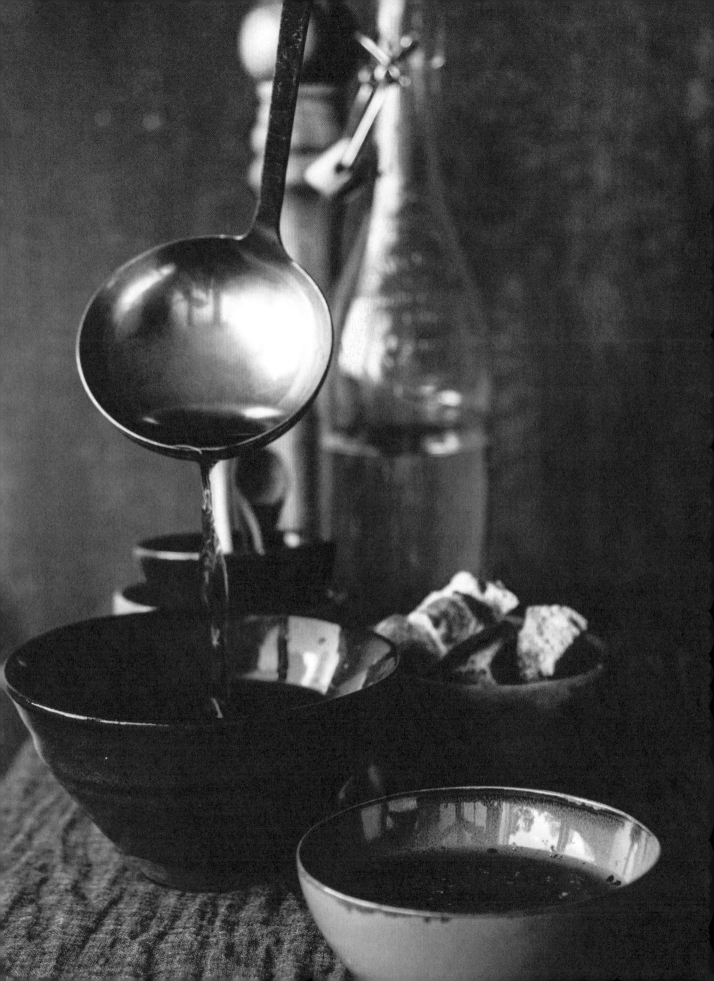

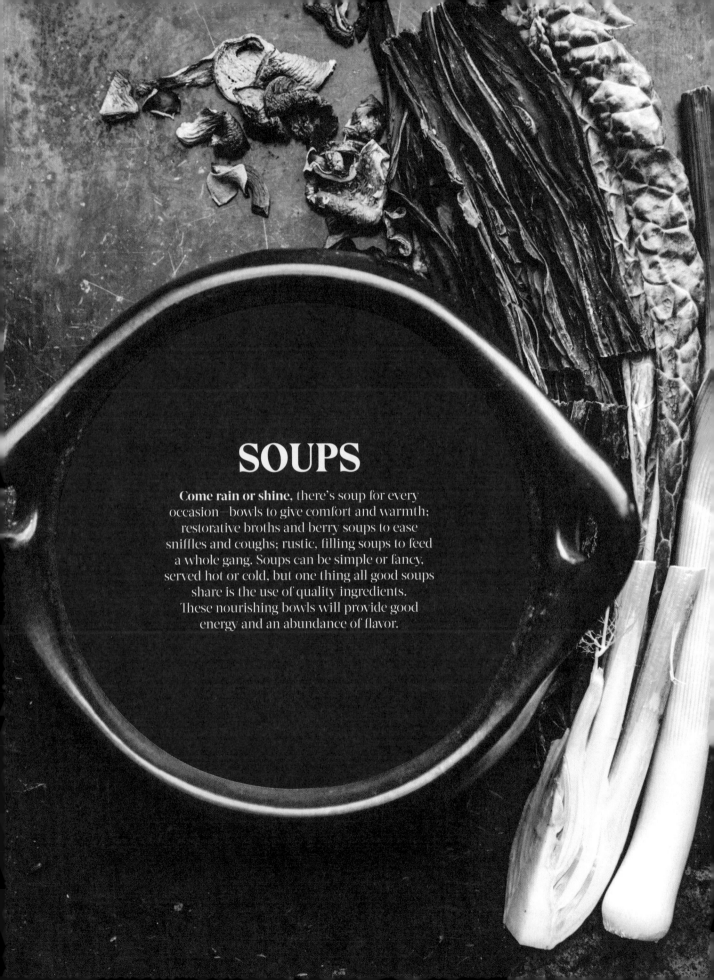

SOUPS

Come rain or shine, there's soup for every occasion—bowls to give comfort and warmth; restorative broths and berry soups to ease sniffles and coughs; rustic, filling soups to feed a whole gang. Soups can be simple or fancy, served hot or cold, but one thing all good soups share is the use of quality ingredients. These nourishing bowls will provide good energy and an abundance of flavor.

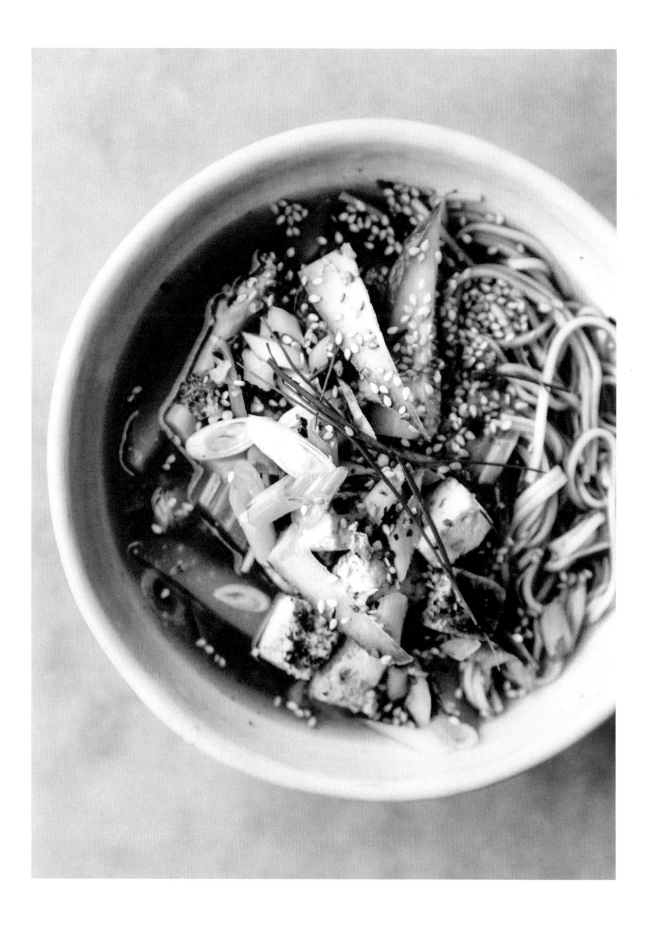

Miso Happy

MISO SOUP WITH GINGER, TOFU, SOBA NOODLES, AND SHIITAKE MUSHROOMS

This easy-to-make soup is the perfect comfort food all year round. Miso is a big deal in Japan where it's a staple of daily life. Its uses are endless and its rich flavor makes it a great addition to any kitchen. Miso paste is made from fermented soybeans and is available in different varieties—lighter miso is milder in taste and has been fermented for less time than the darker variety.

Miso soup is popular for fasting and weight loss as it contains very few calories. It's also a perfect restorative soup when you want to recharge with something light. This recipe delivers the lightness of miso soup while adding a little extra texture and flavor.

To make the dashi, soak the kombu in the water in the fridge for a minimum of 1 hour, preferably overnight. Transfer to a large saucepan, bring to a simmer, then remove the kombu. Strain the liquid through a sieve and refrigerate until ready to use.

Cook the soba noodles according to the package instructions. Rinse in cold water and drain.

Heat a skillet over medium-high heat and add a drizzle of canola oil. Stir-fry the shiitake mushrooms over medium-high heat for a couple of minutes, then remove from the pan. Wipe out the pan and add another drizzle of canola oil, then stir-fry the tofu cubes until golden and sprinkle with salt and a little shichimi togarashi. Remove from the heat.

Bring the dashi to a boil in a large saucepan, then reduce the heat to a simmer. Add the ginger, shoyu, mushrooms, and broccolini and simmer for 10 minutes, then remove from the heat.

Measure out 1 cup of the dashi broth and dissolve the miso in it. Pour the concentrated miso dashi back into the saucepan with the rest of the dashi and add the lime juice and sesame oil. Taste and adjust the flavor with additional miso paste, if needed.

Pour the miso soup into four bowls then add the tofu cubes and soba noodles. Top with cucumber, scallions, and sesame seeds, chives, or cilantro.

VE ✓ GF ✓

SERVES 4

DASHI *(makes 4 cups)*
1 strip of kombu seaweed
4 cups water

MISO SOUP
8 oz. soba noodles
drizzle of canola oil
¼ lb. shiitake mushrooms
5 oz. firm tofu, cut into small cubes
salt
few pinches of shichimi togarashi
    or red pepper flakes
1 tablespoon freshly grated ginger
2 tablespoons shoyu
½ cup broccolini or broccoli florets
4¼ tablespoons miso paste
    (I use white or yellow)
juice of ½ lime
drizzle of sesame oil

TOPPINGS
cucumber, cut into matchsticks
2 scallions, thinly sliced
handful of sesame seeds
handful of fresh herbs (chives or
    cilantro fit perfectly)

Dhal Tadka

CREAM OF RED LENTILS WITH AN ALMOND AND ONION TADKA

This dish amazes me every time. To think that plain cooked lentils have so much taste astounds me. Dhal means soup in Sanskrit and is India's number one comfort meal.

There are plenty of reasons to love this humble meal. It's delicious, healthy, and easy to make! The first rule of making a dhal is to allow sufficient time for simmering the legumes into a creamy soup. The longer they have to break down, the silkier the dhal. Pre-soaking helps the softening process.

The lentils are flavored by tadka, which is a tempered spice mix. Enjoy with raita (see page 133) and naan bread for a more substantial meal.

Put the lentils into a large saucepan with the water. Bring to a boil and skim off any foam that rises to the surface with a spoon. Boil the lentils for 35 to 50 minutes, adding more water if it starts to dry up. Keep adding water to achieve the desired consistency. When the lentils are dissolved and creamy, remove the pan from the heat.

To make the tadka, heat a saucepan over medium heat and add 2 tablespoons ghee or coconut oil. Sauté the shallots, garlic, and almonds over low heat until the shallots are golden and translucent. The shallots should sweat and release their juices rather than getting crisp. Add another tablespoon of ghee or coconut oil with the rest of the tadka ingredients and stir-fry for another 3 minutes before removing from the heat.

Reserve a small amount of the tadka for garnish and blend the rest of the mixture to a smooth paste with a few tablespoons water. Before serving, bring the dhal to a simmer and mix in the tadka. Remove from the heat and serve with fresh cilantro and the reserved tadka. You can make this a bigger meal by adding raita and naan bread.

VE *Use coconut oil instead of ghee.*

GF *Serve with gluten-free bread instead of naan bread.*

GHEE THAT'S GOOD! *Ghee is a type of clarified butter that originated in India. It's highly regarded in holistic and Ayurvedic teachings. With a high smoke point, ghee makes a healthy choice for frying and cooking at high temperatures. Use ghee where you would butter and it will give a more intense flavor. Ghee is not vegan—use quality coconut oil as a substitute.*

SERVES 4 TO 6
2 cups red lentils or yellow split peas or mung beans, soaked and drained if you have time
6 cups water

TADKA SPICE MIX
3 tablespoons ghee or coconut oil
4 shallots, finely sliced
3 garlic cloves, finely sliced
1 tablespoon ground almonds
juice of 1 lime
1 tablespoon tomato paste
1 teaspoon freshly grated or ground turmeric
3/4 teaspoon salt
1 teaspoon ground cumin
1 teaspoon mustard seeds
1 teaspoon freshly grated ginger
1 teaspoon ground coriander
1/2 red chile pepper (or more to taste), finely chopped
1 teaspoon coconut sugar

TO SERVE
fresh cilantro
raita (optional, see page 133)
naan (optional)

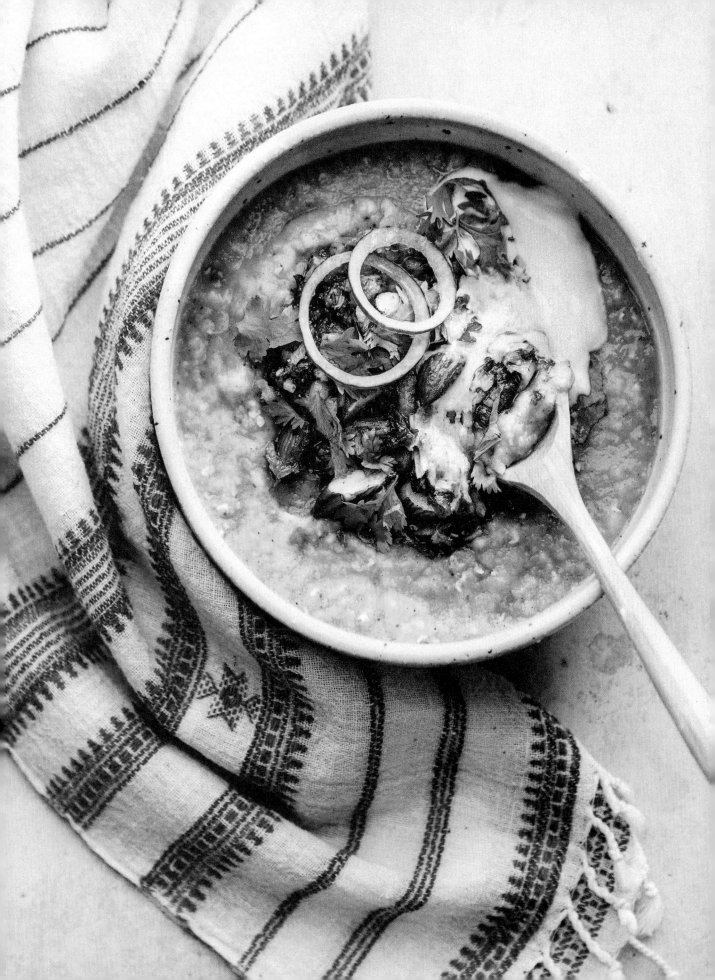

A Very Green Soup

GREEN PEA AND SPINACH QUINOA WITH WASABI CREAM

This chlorophyll-rich soup with peas and spinach is filled with light energy—a perfect reboot dish when you need a fresh start. The quinoa gives a little more body and boosts the nutrition with extra protein as well as adding a pleasing texture. Quinoa needs a little longer to cook than the rest of the ingredients, so I prepare it beforehand to keep the cooking time for the peas and spinach really short and to allow them to retain maximum freshness. To preserve their flavors, the basil and mint are only added after removing the soup from the heat—all in the name of vibrant taste! Drizzle with the wasabi cream for a perfect finish.

Cook the quinoa according to the package instructions. Drain and set aside. Mix the ingredients for the wasabi cream, then cover and refrigerate until ready to serve.

Melt the coconut oil in a saucepan over medium-low heat. Add the sliced shallots and celery. Salt and pepper lightly, then toss and stir until the shallots are translucent, about 5 minutes.

Pour in the vegetable broth and bring to a boil. Add the peas, spinach, ginger, garlic, and cooked quinoa and simmer for 2 minutes. Remove from the heat before adding the mint, basil, and olive oil. Blend to a smooth consistency or leave some texture if you prefer. Taste and adjust the seasoning with salt and pepper and serve with wasabi cream.

Tip! Get creative and swap the wasabi edge in the sauce for horseradish or mustard—the brave can increase the measures for a harder hit.

VE *Use maple or agave syrup instead of honey, and use vegan crème fraîche (see page 50).*

GF ✓

SERVES 4

¾ cups quinoa
3 tablespoons coconut oil
3 shallots, sliced
1 celery stalk, sliced
4 cups vegetable broth (see page 56)
1 lb. green peas
¾ lb. spinach, roughly chopped
½ tablespoon freshly grated ginger
1 garlic clove, finely chopped
handful of mint leaves
handful of basil leaves
extra-virgin olive oil
salt and pepper

WASABI CREAM

¾ cup vegan crème fraîche (see page 50) or dairy crème fraîche
½ tablespoon wasabi (or more for a stronger taste)
2 tablespoons extra-virgin olive oil
1 teaspoon honey or agave syrup
juice of ¼ lemon

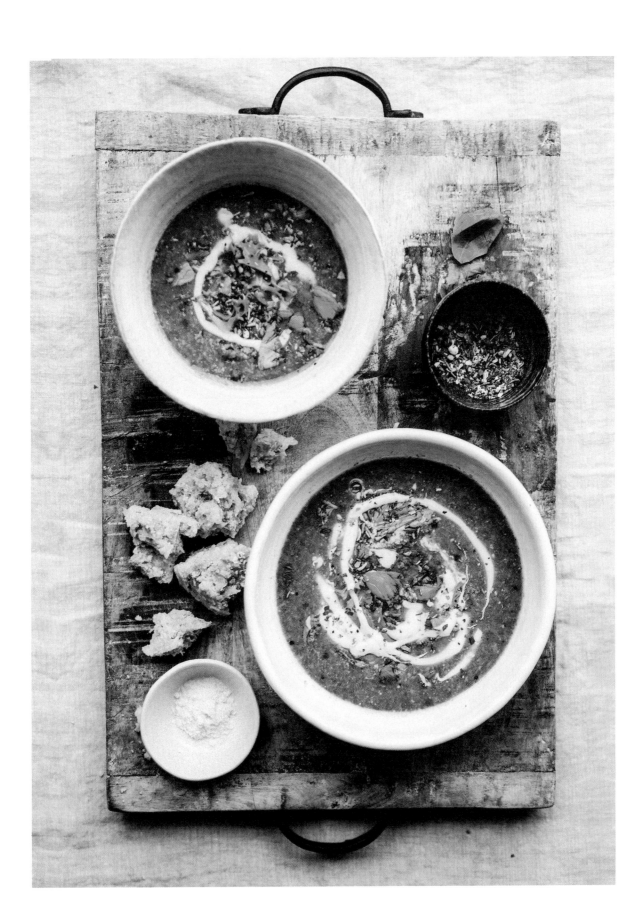

Yogisha Soup

SWEET POTATO, CILANTRO, AND COCONUT SOUP

Not all relationships last, but favorite dishes can provide lifelong enjoyment. An ex-boyfriend's mum who was a yoga teacher often made this soup, and we both shared a love for healthy dishes with Indian and Ayurvedic influences. We would delight in this gentle soup, which always tastes nourishing and comforting—it's like a big hug in a bowl. After the relationship with my boyfriend ended, I kept his mum's soup as a regular dish. Over the years I varied the recipe many times; it started out as a carrot soup and I currently like to make it with the addition of sweet potato. It's a real keeper.

Melt the coconut oil in a saucepan over medium-low heat and sauté the shallots until translucent. Add the carrots, sweet potato, ginger, garlic, ground coriander, cayenne, and a little salt. Stir-fry for 3 to 4 minutes before adding the vegetable broth, coconut milk, salt, and kaffir lime leaves. Simmer until the sweet potato is soft and tender, about 15 minutes.

Remove from the heat and discard the lime leaves. Add the fresh cilantro and blend until silky smooth. Taste and adjust the seasoning with salt and pepper. Serve sprinkled with hemp seeds.

VE ✓ GF ✓

SERVES 4

1–2 tablespoons coconut oil
3 large shallots, finely sliced
1 lb. carrots, finely sliced
1 lb. sweet potatoes, peeled and cut into small cubes
2 tablespoon freshly grated ginger
2 garlic cloves, finely chopped to a paste
1 tablespoon ground coriander
$\frac{1}{4}$ teaspoon cayenne pepper
3 cups vegetable broth (see page 56)
14 oz. can coconut milk
$\frac{3}{4}$ tablespoon salt
3–4 kaffir lime leaves
bunch of fresh cilantro, roughly chopped
salt and pepper

TO SERVE
hemp seeds

AYURVEDIC COOKING! *Ayurveda is an ancient Hindu system of natural medicine that developed from the Vedic scriptures (which also gave rise to yoga). Ayurvedic cooking seeks balance and harmony by assessing individual nourishment needs. The goal is to eat for a healthy body and a clear mind with free-flowing energies. An Ayurvedic diet can prescribe energizing or calming foods, or foods that activate the digestive system.*

Ayurvedic cooking is a holistic approach to health that takes your whole life into account. Restoring balance often means adding a contrast that's been missing. If you're curious about Ayurveda, consult an Ayurvedic practitioner for dietary advice.

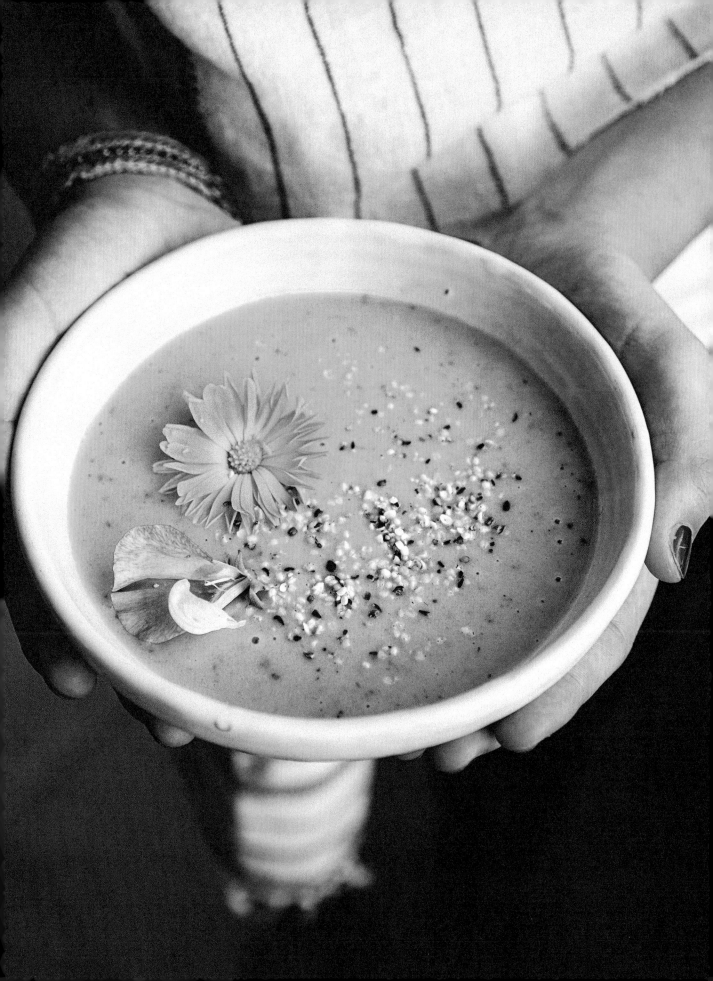

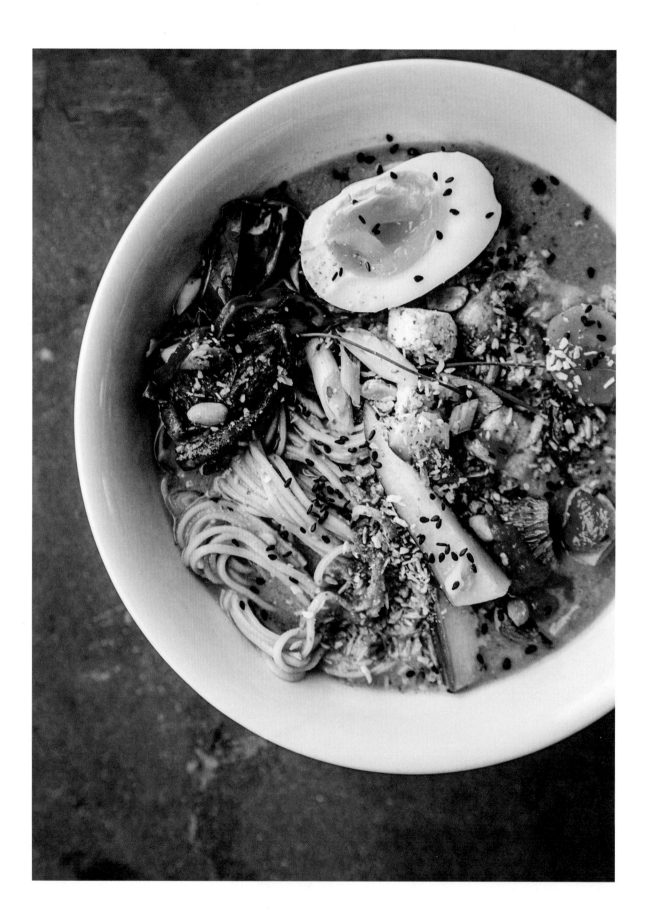

Ramen Wonder

SOBA NOODLES IN SPICY RAMEN BROTH

This recipe is a real gem, a deliciously healthy ramen noodle soup bowl. Ramen noodles are the Andy Warhol of food these days! What started as a cheap post-war budget dish in Japan is now a worldwide phenomenon. It's easy to understand why: the creativity involved in making a good ramen fuses the authentic food traditions of Asia with the rest of the world.

The key to a perfect ramen bowl lies in using quality broth, which requires patience and time—up to two days for some recipes. I've put together this ramen recipe so that you can make the most delicious savory ramen soup in no time. If you already have prepared dashi (page 39) or vegetable broth (page 56) it's done in a flash. If you need to make dashi or vegetable broth, factor in an additional hour. The real flavor punch comes from the tare—a spice mixture dissolved into the broth.

In the spirit of ramen, I fused Japanese ingredients with flavors from other world kitchens. Mixing soy sauce, tamarind, miso, tahini, and Sriracha makes this bowl full of flavor. Toppings are optional, but a mixture of fresh raw vegetables such as carrot, cucumber, and avocado makes a beautiful pairing with the savory shiitake mushrooms, chives, and eggs. Try adding a crisp crunch with toasted coconut flakes and peanuts (seroendeng).

Pour the dashi or vegetable broth into a large saucepan. Bring to a boil over medium-high heat. Add the dried shiitake mushrooms and vegetables to the broth with a pinch of salt. Lower the heat and let the broth simmer until ready to assemble.

Transfer 1 cup of strained dashi or broth to a small saucepan. Bring to a boil, then reduce to a simmer. Add the tare ingredients and blend in a food processor until smooth. Simmer over low heat until ready to serve.

Prepare the add-ins and toppings and cook the noodles according to the package instructions. Rinse the noodles in cold water and set aside. Pour the remaining vegetable broth into serving bowls. Stir the tare mixture into the broth. Divide the drained noodles, add-ins, and toppings between the bowls. Customize your heat and strength of flavor. Serve with condiments like Sriracha, soy sauce, and toasted sesame oil.

VE *Omit the eggs. If you purchase dashi, check it's a vegan product, as commercial dashi is often made with bonito flakes (dried tuna).*

GF *Use soba or other gluten-free noodles. Use gluten-free tamari instead of soy sauce.*

SERVES 4

5 cups dashi (see page 39) or vegetable broth (see page 56)
handful of dried shiitake mushrooms
1–1½ lbs. mixed soup vegetables (like sliced carrots and broccoli florets)
pinch of salt
8 oz. soba or ramen noodles

TARE

2 tablespoons miso paste (I used yellow)
¼ cup soy sauce
¼ cup mirin
5 garlic cloves, crushed
1½ tablespoons Sriracha
3 tablespoons chickpea flour
1½ tablespoons tahini
1 tablespoon toasted sesame oil
1 tablespoon tamarind paste
½ tablespoon freshly grated ginger

ADD-INS (OPTIONAL)

½ lb. shiitake mushrooms, fried
3.5 oz. tofu, fried
½ cucumber, cut into matchsticks
5 scallions, sliced
pickles (I used pickled red cabbage)
4 medium eggs, boiled and halved
1 cup seroendeng, optional, (mix ½ cup desiccated coconut with ½ cup crushed peanuts and toast in a skillet for 1½ minutes)

TOPPINGS

handful of chives, handful of black sesame seeds, sprinkling of shichimi togarashi or red pepper flakes, pickles

Fish-Free Bouillabaisse

RUSTIC SAFFRON AND VEGETABLE SOUP WITH SEAWEED AND ROUILLE

There's something very romantic about rustic soups such as bouillabaisse. As much as I like perfectly blended soups, the sense of the Old World that derives from a soup full of texture is hard to beat. This one comes from Marseilles, the old seaport in southern France. In this recipe I have transformed what was originally a fish stew into a delicious vegetarian soup, infusing it with a seafood flavor from kombu seaweed.

A traditional bouillabaisse is made with a variety of seafood, often the leftovers after fishermen have sold the best of their catch. To duplicate the various textures in a classic bouillabaisse I used a mixture of vegetables, giving cauliflower a prominent position. The soup's flavor is elevated by saffron, fennel, and almond. It is served with a tasty rouille sauce made with roasted pepper and mayonnaise, which is spooned into the finished soup and scooped up with bread.

Preheat the oven to 400°F and line a baking sheet with parchment. Place the peppers, sweet potato, and cauliflower florets on the baking sheet. Drizzle with olive oil and sprinkle with salt and thyme. Roast until soft, about 30 minutes. Remove from the oven and set aside. Once cool enough to handle, peel the skin from the whole red pepper, then halve and remove seeds, ready to make the rouille.

Blend all the ingredients for the rouille and refrigerate, covered, until ready to serve.

To make the soup, heat a saucepan over medium-high heat and add a drizzle of olive oil. Gently cook the garlic, fennel, shallots, and almonds for a few minutes. Add the leek and cook, stirring, for a another minute. Add the broth, tomatoes, wine, kombu, bay leaves, olives, nutritional yeast (if using), honey, and ½ teaspoon salt. Cover the pan and let it simmer slowly for 15 minutes. Add the roasted vegetables, chickpeas, and saffron, then continue to simmer for 10 minutes.

Remove from heat and discard the kombu and bay leaves. Add the Pernod (if using), and salt and pepper to taste. Drizzle with extra-virgin olive oil and serve with the rouille and rustic bread.

VE *Use Vegenaise for the rouille and maple or agave syrup instead of honey.*

GF *Serve with gluten-free bread.*

SERVES 2 TO 3

2 red bell peppers, 1 cut into strips and 1 left whole
1 sweet potato, peeled and cut into ½-inch dice
2 cups cauliflower florets
olive oil
2 tablespoons fresh thyme
4 garlic cloves, sliced
1 fennel bulb, thinly sliced
3 shallots, thinly sliced
handful of almonds, thinly sliced
½ leek, thinly sliced
4 cups vegetable broth (see page 56)
14½ oz. can diced tomatoes
⅔ cup dry white wine
4-inch strip of kombu seaweed
2 bay leaves
¼ lb. black olives
3 tablespoons nutritional yeast (optional)
1 teaspoon honey or maple syrup
8 oz. can chickpeas, drained
1 saffron thread
1 tablespoon Pernod (optional)
salt and pepper
extra-virgin olive oil

ROUILLE

1 red bell pepper, roasted (see above)
½ cup mayonnaise or Vegenaise
juice of 1 lemon
2 garlic cloves, crushed
pinch of ground star anise (optional)
½ teaspoon harissa paste
salt

rustic bread, to serve

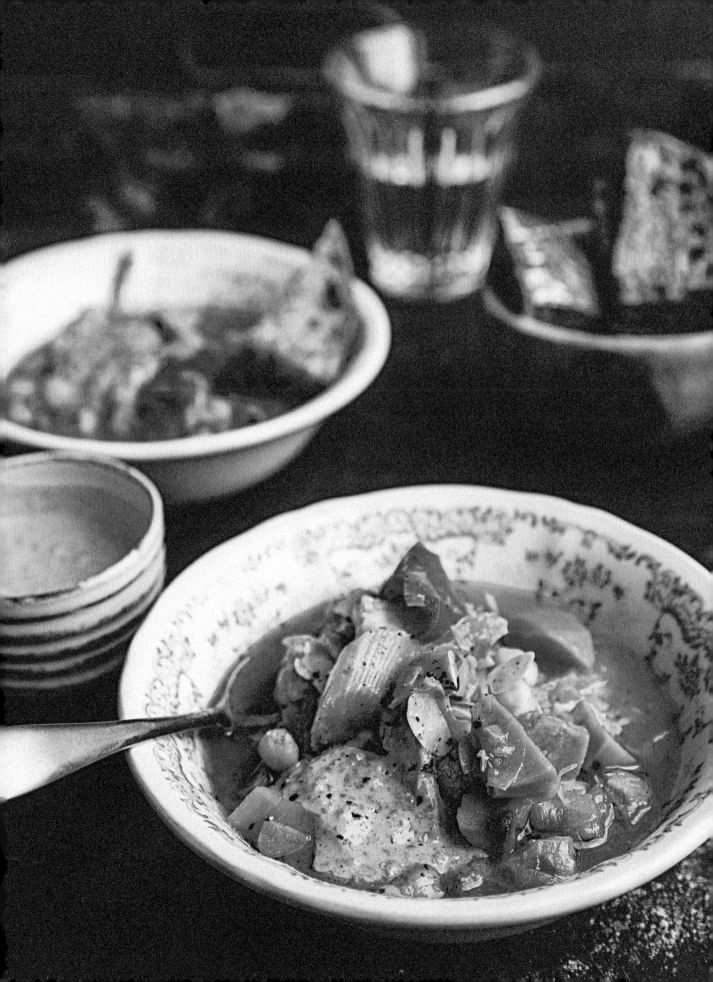

Eggplant and Pepper Soup

CREAM OF ROASTED EGGPLANT AND PEPPER WITH THYME AND LEMON FRAÎCHE

Roasting vegetables releases deeply satisfying flavors. Eggplant, a rather dull vegetable when raw, is transformed into a mouthwatering delicacy after a turn in the oven! Blending roasted eggplant with the sweet juices of roasted peppers and tomatoes makes an irresistible soup with distinct Mediterranean flavors. For a beautiful contrast, serve hot with a swirl of crème fraîche.

Preheat the oven to 400°F and line a baking sheet with parchment. If you are making vegan crème fraîche, blend the ingredients, adding a little water at a time until you achieve the desired consistency. Refrigerate until ready to serve.

To make the soup, place the eggplants, tomatoes, and peppers cut side up on the lined sheet. Drizzle with olive oil and sprinkle with salt and thyme. Roast for 45 minutes.

Meanwhile, heat a drizzle of olive oil in a saucepan and slowly cook the shallots, garlic, and walnuts over medium heat for 5 minutes. Sprinkle with salt and place in a food processor with the roasted veggies, tahini, paprika, and a third of the broth. Blend until smooth. Pour the soup back into the saucepan and stir in the rest of the vegetable stock and the lemon juice. Bring to a boil, then remove from heat. Taste and adjust the seasoning with salt and pepper. Drizzle in a little extra-virgin olive oil. Serve with crème fraîche, Parmesan, and basil.

Tip! This soup can also be served cold, like gazpacho.

VE *Use vegan crème fraîche and rawmesan instead of Parmesan. Or omit the cheese and crème fraîche entirely.*

GF ✓

SERVES 3 TO 4

2 eggplants, halved
½ lb. cherry tomatoes, halved
4 red bell peppers, halved, seeded, and cut into pieces
olive oil
leave from several sprigs of thyme
5 shallots, finely diced
2–3 garlic cloves, finely minced
handful of walnuts, crushed
2 tablespoons tahini
1 teaspoon paprika
4 cups vegetable broth (see page 56)
juice of 1 lemon
extra-virgin olive oil
salt and pepper

TO SERVE (OPTIONAL)

crème fraîche (see recipe for vegan version below)
grated Parmesan or rawmesan (see page 53)
fresh basil

VEGAN CRÈME FRAÎCHE

1 cup raw cashews, soaked overnight and drained
juice of 1 lemon
pinch of salt
1 teaspoon extra-virgin olive oil

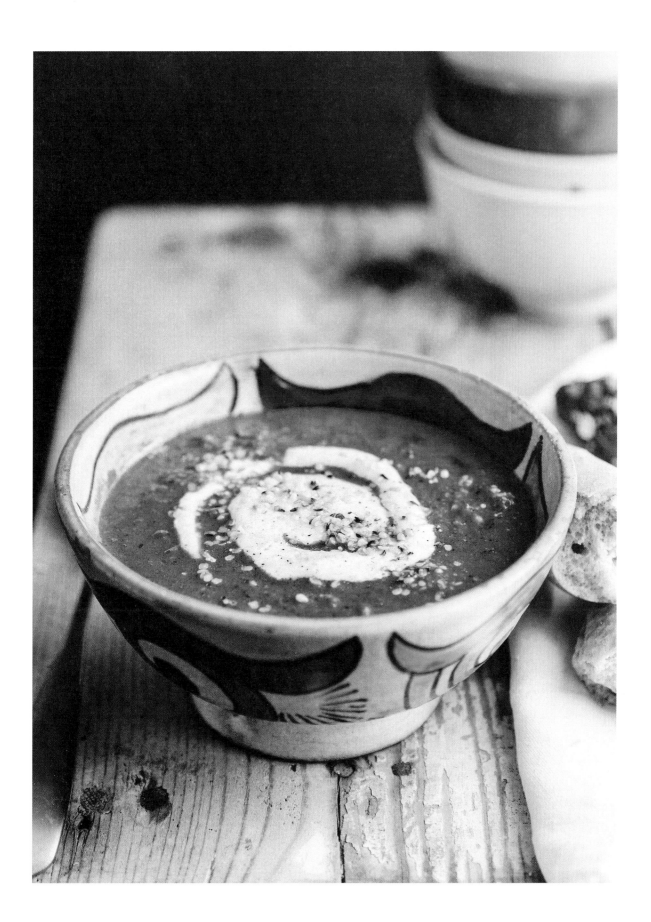

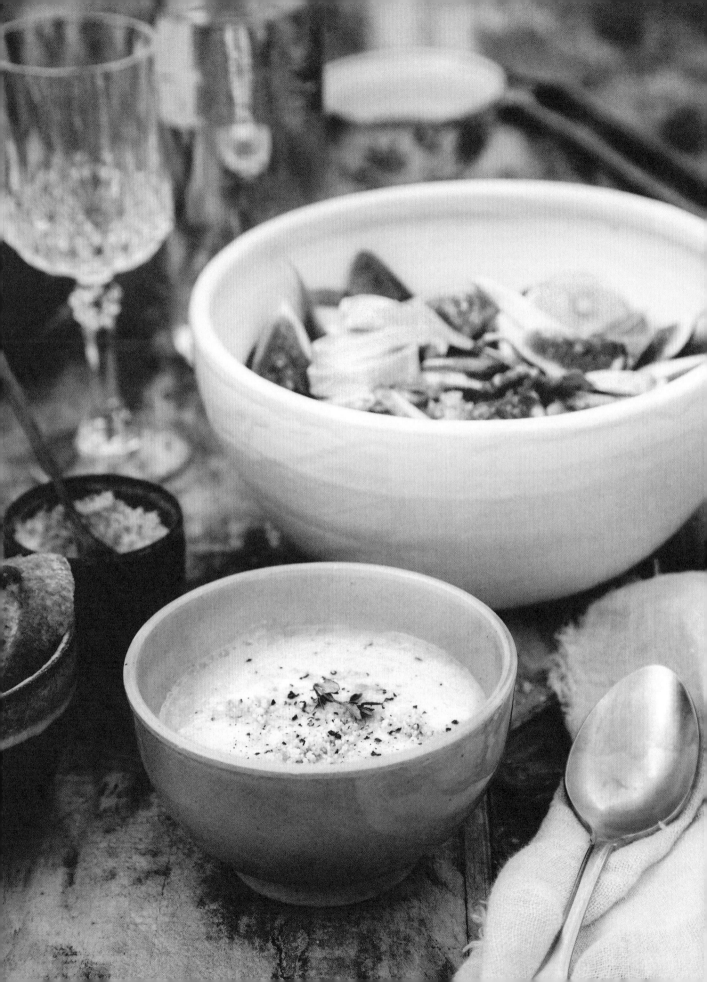

Sunchoke Soup

A CREAMY JERUSALEM ARTICHOKE SOUP WITH PROSECCO, THYME, AND RAWMESAN

I often return to this velvety soup for its beautiful flavor. Sunchokes, also known as Jerusalem artichokes, are an exciting alternative to potatoes and just as versatile, being delicious sautéed, roasted, or puréed. In this soup, their nutty sweet flavor is complemented by tangy lemon and Prosecco. If you're making this soup for dinner guests, topping it with roasted choke crisps and Parmesan will add to the refined look and taste. I like to alternate Parmesan with a so-called rawmesan—a mixture of nutritional yeast and crumbled nuts—which is a delicious vegan alternative to grated cheese.

First make the crisps. Preheat the oven to 300°F and line a baking sheet with parchment. Spread the sunchoke slices on the lined sheet and sprinkle with salt. Bake until golden, about 15 minutes, keeping an eye on the crisps to make sure they don't burn. Remove from the oven and set aside to cool.

Meanwhile make the rawmesan. Roughly blend or grind all the ingredients. Set aside in a covered bowl until ready to serve (it keeps for a week in the fridge).

For the soup, put a large saucepan over medium-high heat. Melt the coconut oil, add the shallots, and stir-fry for 1 to 2 minutes. Add the garlic and thyme and cook 1 to 2 minutes more. Add the sunchokes, with more oil if needed, and cook for 1 minute, stirring well. Pour the broth, coconut milk, and Prosecco into the pan. Add the honey, salt, and black pepper. Let simmer over medium heat for 15 to 18 minutes.

Remove the soup from the heat and blend until smooth. Use a sieve to sift the chickpea flour, if using, into the soup, then blend well. Stir in the lemon juice and olive oil. Taste and adjust the seasoning with salt and pepper. Serve with Parmesan or rawmesan and top with the crisps.

Tip! Make a big batch of the crisps so you can enjoy them with Netflix later!

VE *Use rawmesan instead of Parmesan and agave syrup instead of honey. Use coconut oil instead of butter.*

GF *Choose gluten-free bread.*

SERVES 2 TO 3 AS A MAIN
COURSE OR 4 AS A STARTER

1 tablespoon coconut oil or butter
2 shallots, finely chopped
2 garlic cloves, finely chopped
1½ tablespoons fresh thyme leaves
1–1½ lbs. sunchokes (Jerusalem artichokes), peeled and diced
1–2 cups vegetable broth (see page 56)
14 oz. can coconut milk
¾ cup Prosecco
1 teaspoon honey or agave syrup
1 teaspoon salt
black pepper
3 tablespoons chickpea flour (optional)
juice of ¼ lemon
2 tablespoons extra-virgin olive oil

CRISPS FOR TOPPING

1 or more Jerusalem artichokes, scrubbed and sliced into thin rounds
salt

RAWMESAN

2 tablespoons hemp seeds (optional)
2 tablespoons nutritional yeast
¾ cup pine nuts
½ teaspoon salt
drizzle of lemon juice

White Gazpacho

CHILLED CUCUMBER, AVOCADO, GINGER, AND COCONUT SOUP

During hot summer days, I find myself craving ice-cold juices, fresh smoothies, and chilled soups. This cool cucumber and coconut soup is just right when the weather is warm and you want a refreshing, light meal. Inspired by Spanish gazpacho, it has Asian accents of lime, ginger, cilantro, and sesame seed oil. Avocado and cucumber are heavenly with the more savory notes of garlic and toasted sesame seeds. Make a double batch and keep in the fridge as a refreshment for up to two days.

Heat a skillet over medium-high heat and add the coconut oil. Cook the garlic, shallots, celery, yellow pepper, chile pepper, scallions, and ginger until the shallots are translucent and the vegetables are tender. Cool, then transfer to a blender.

Add the diced cucumber and avocado with the rest of the soup ingredients to the blender and process until smooth. Taste and adjust the seasoning with salt. Pour into a pitcher or decanter and chill for at least 20 minutes.

Serve in bowls topped with scallion, sesame seeds, and lime zest and drizzle with a little swirl of sesame oil.

VE ✓
GF *Use gluten-free tamari instead of soy sauce.*

SERVES 2
1 tablespoon coconut oil
2 garlic cloves, finely chopped
2 shallots, finely chopped
1 celery stalk, finely sliced
½ yellow bell pepper, seeded and diced
½ red chile pepper, seeded, and finely chopped
4 scallions, sliced
¾ teaspoon freshly grated ginger
1 medium cucumber, diced
1 avocado, pitted, peeled, and diced
juice and zest of 1 lime
2 (14 oz.) cans coconut milk
¼ cup soy sauce
handful of fresh cilantro
handful of fresh mint
salt

TOPPINGS
1 scallion, finely chopped
toasted sesame seeds
lime zest
toasted sesame oil

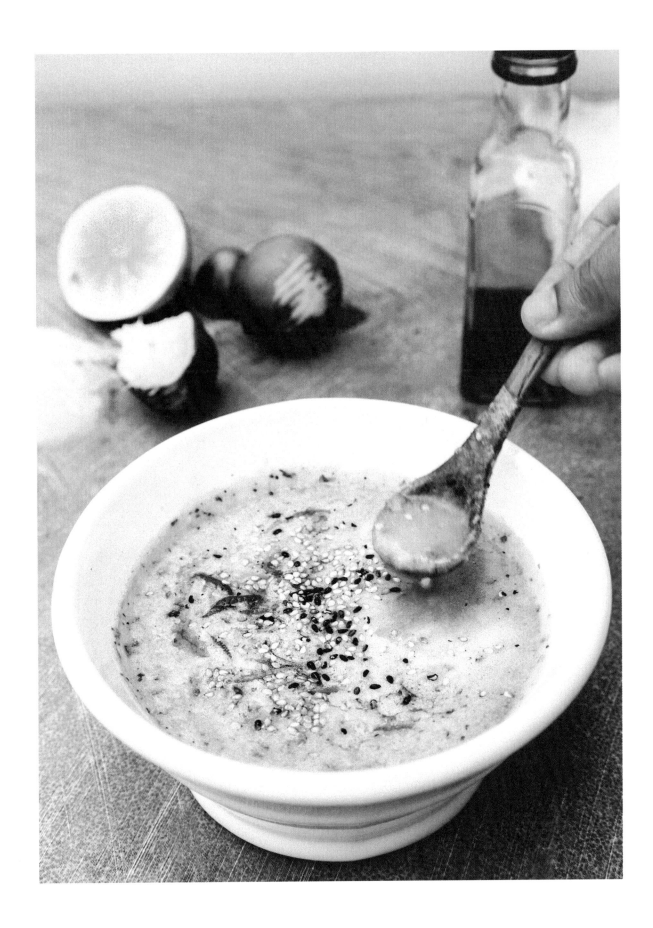

Vegetable Broth

BECAUSE YOU WANT TO MAKE YOUR OWN

Making your own broth can seem more complicated than it is. In fact, it's incredibly easy and pays huge dividends in taste. It's also the perfect opportunity to avoid waste because any vegetables you know you won't finish before they spoil can go into the pot. Onions are great for flavor, as are celery stalks. Take your broth to the next level by adding roasted vegetables, mushrooms, and more defining flavors such as ginger, garlic, and spices. Just remember not to add salt—or salty ingredients such as soy sauce—until it's time to use the broth in a soup or other dish. For Asian soup bases, use the recipe for Japanese dashi (see page 39).

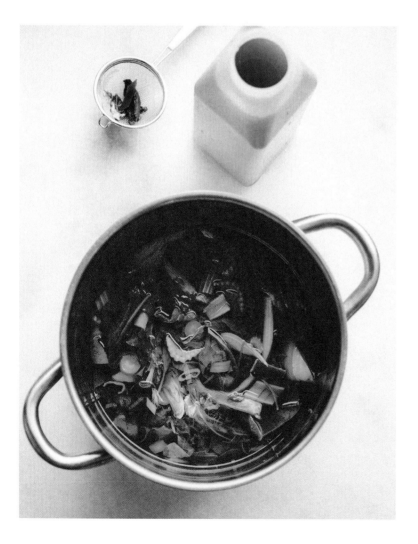

BASIC VEGETABLE BROTH
mix of root vegetables like celery, carrot, and leek, washed and chopped
onions
water, to cover

NEXT-LEVEL VEGETABLE BROTH
add-ins to the basic broth
handful of dried mushrooms
roasted vegetables (squash and root vegetables like beets, potato, carrot, parsnip, onions)
bay leaves
herbs
kaffir lime leaves
ginger
garlic
peppers

Cover the vegetables with water. Bring to a boil and lower the heat. Let the broth simmer for 45 minutes to 1 hour. Remove the vegetables with a slotted spoon. Filter the broth through a fine sieve or a colander lined with cheesecloth. Freeze the broth in tightly sealed containers until ready to use. It keeps for at least a month in the freezer.

VE ✓ GF ✓

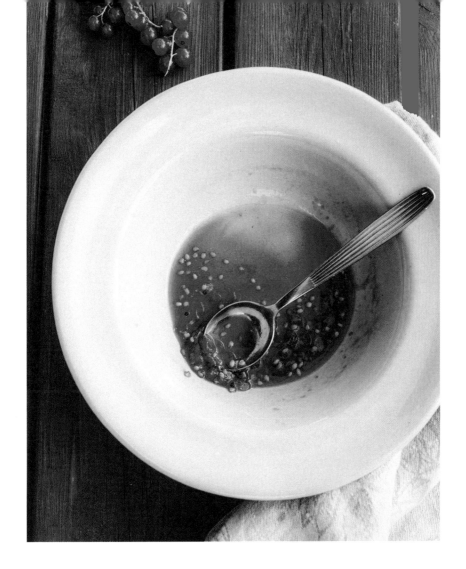

Red Currant Remedy Soup

COLD-PRESSED RED CURRANT SOUP

This cold-fighting soup is made by cold-pressing red currants, which preserves their powerful vitamins. The sour berries are sweetened by manuka honey, renowned for its antibacterial properties. Eaten cold, this soup is also very tasty when you're not ill, and can be served as a healthier dessert with yogurt or ice cream.

2½ cups fresh red currants
juice of 1 lemon
1½ tablespoons manuka honey
almond milk (optional)

Clean the red currants and remove the stems. Add to a bowl with the lemon. Mash the berries with a mashing tool (as you would use for potatoes) and mix in the honey. Serve as is or with a splash of almond milk and eat immediately.

VE *Use agave or maple syrup instead of manuka honey.*

GF ✓

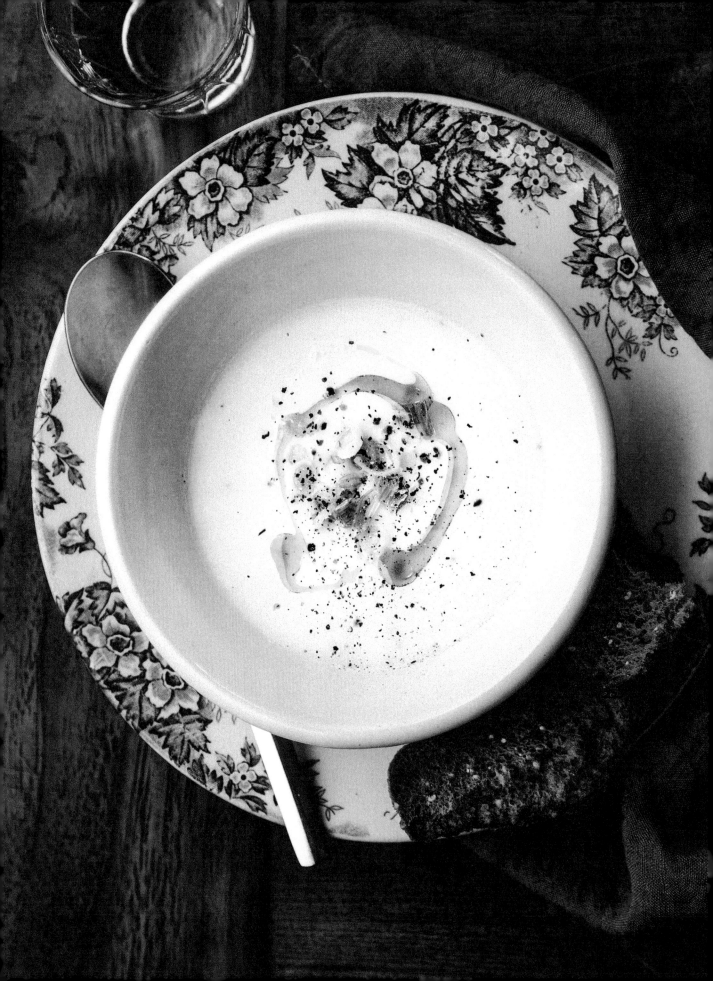

Leek Soup

CREAMY POTATO AND LEEK SOUP

This comforting and filling potato and leek soup is always a hit! The leeks give it a wonderful flavor and the potatoes add substance. If you prefer, you can substitute Jerusalem artichokes for the potatoes. This soup is based on the classic French Vichyssoise, but tweaked by replacing the heavy cream with the lighter creaminess of almond milk, almond butter, and crème fraîche. Use vegan crème fraîche to make it completely plant-based.

Boil the potatoes in a large saucepan until soft, then drain and set aside. Heat a drizzle of olive oil or 2 tablespoons butter in a skillet over medium-high heat and sauté the leeks until soft, 2 to 3 minutes.

In a large saucepan, combine the leeks with the potatoes and the remaining soup ingredients and bring to a boil. Reduce the heat to low and let it simmer for 10 minutes. Remove from the heat, transfer to a food processor, and blend until smooth. Serve with bread and a drizzle of extra-virgin olive oil.

Tip! This soup can be served cold or warm; the traditional Vichyssoise soup is often served cold.

VE *Use olive oil instead of butter and vegan crème fraîche.*

GF *Serve with gluten-free bread.*

SERVES 4

1 lb. russet potatoes, peeled and diced
drizzle of olive oil or 2 tablespoons butter
5 leeks, cleaned and cut into pieces
3 cups vegetable broth (see page 56)
1½ cups almond milk
¼ cup white wine
2 tablespoons almond butter
⅓ cup dairy crème fraîche or vegan crème fraîche
1 teaspoon salt
black pepper

TO SERVE
bread
extra-virgin olive oil

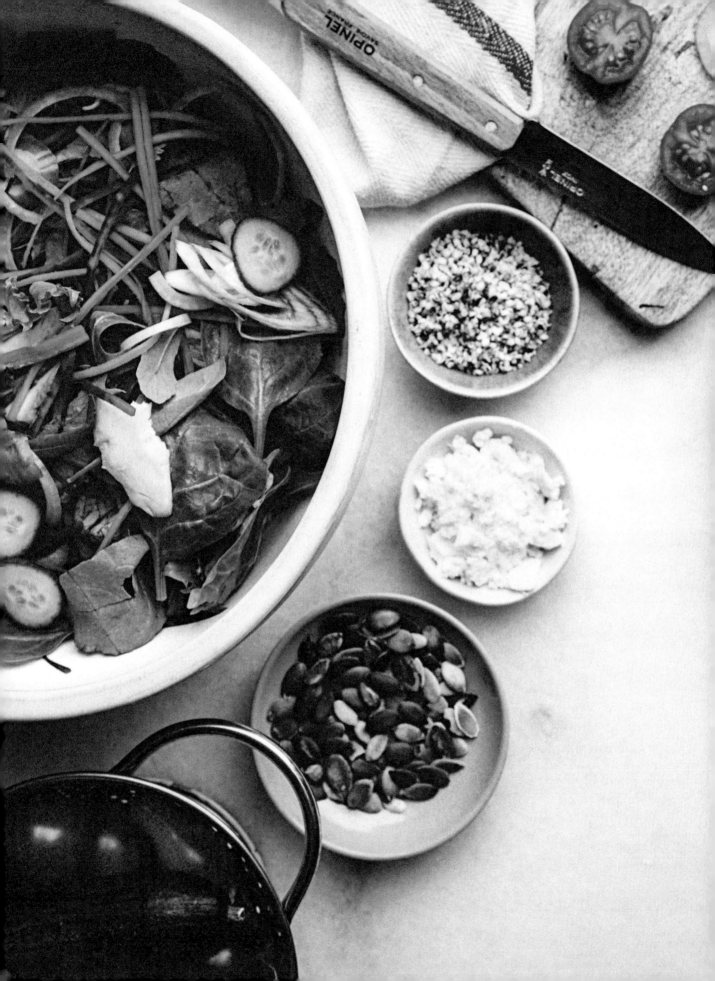

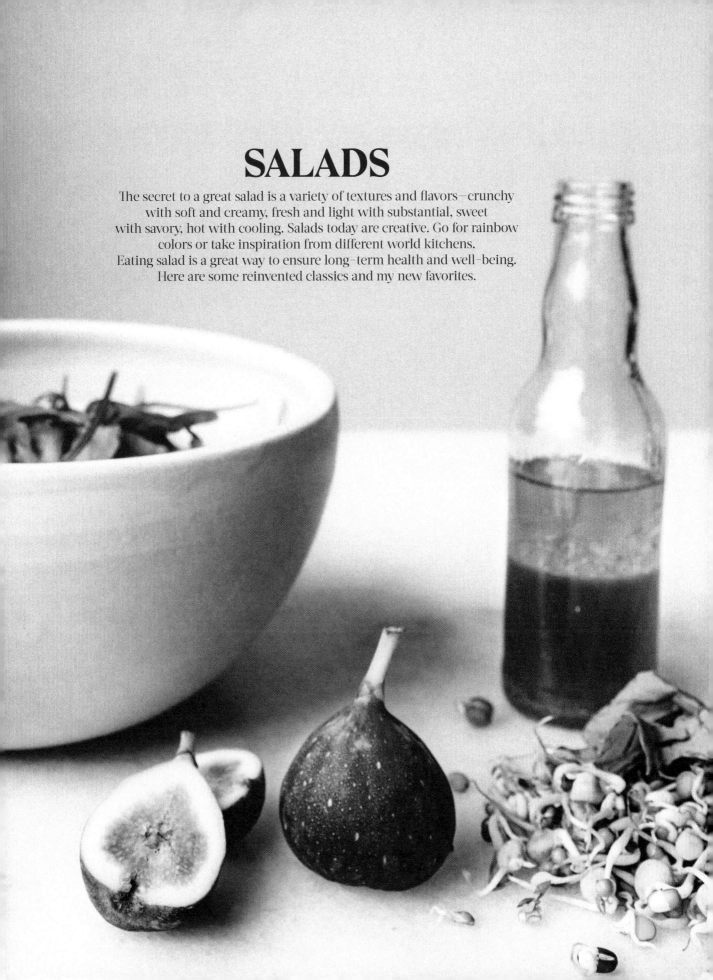

SALADS

The secret to a great salad is a variety of textures and flavors—crunchy
with soft and creamy, fresh and light with substantial, sweet
with savory, hot with cooling. Salads today are creative. Go for rainbow
colors or take inspiration from different world kitchens.
Eating salad is a great way to ensure long-term health and well-being.
Here are some reinvented classics and my new favorites.

Ruby Salad

TOMATOES, PLUMS, AND STRAWBERRIES WITH FETA AND PISTACHIOS

The juices of raw tomatoes, plums, watermelon, and strawberries are in cahoots with each other in this salad, making this bowl a ruby-red beauty with a sweet and savory flavor. Layer with crumbled feta and top with pistachios and pumpkin seeds for a crunchy finish.

You don't need to follow the recipe strictly, just seek out the most vibrant red and purple fruit and vegetables you can find at the farmers market or in your local supermarket. Choose organic feta if you can.

Wash and trim the vegetables, fruit, and berries as needed. Mix the ingredients for the vinaigrette, seasoning with salt and pepper to taste. Cover and set aside.

Heat a skillet over medium-high heat. Toast the pumpkin seeds for a few minutes until they are crisp and golden. Transfer to a small bowl and sprinkle with salt.

Assemble the salad in four serving bowls, starting with the leaves and shredded cabbage, and topping with the rest of the salad ingredients. Drizzle with the vinaigrette and sprinkle with salt. Top with the pumpkin seeds, pistachios, and feta.

Tip! For a more filling salad, add cooked lentils to each serving.

VE *Omit the feta or use vegan nut cheese instead (see page 155).*
GF ✓

SERVES 4
¼ small red cabbage, finely shredded
1–2 red onions, sliced in rounds
½ lb. heirloom tomatoes, halved or quartered according to size
bunch of interesting red leaves, like radicchio or red mesclun
½ lb. watermelon, cut into bite-size pieces
bunch of small red plums, halved, pitted, and cut in wedges
bunch of strawberries or other berries—blueberries, raspberries, blackberries
2 handfuls pumpkin seeds
2 handfuls pistachios, roughly chopped
4 oz. soft feta, crumbled
salt and pepper

HONEY LEMON VINAIGRETTE
½ cup extra-virgin olive oil
2 tablespoons red wine vinegar
juice of 1 lemon
1 tablespoon honey or agave syrup
1 garlic clove, finely chopped to a paste
salt and pepper

OPTIONAL
4 cups cooked firm lentils (Le Puy or black)

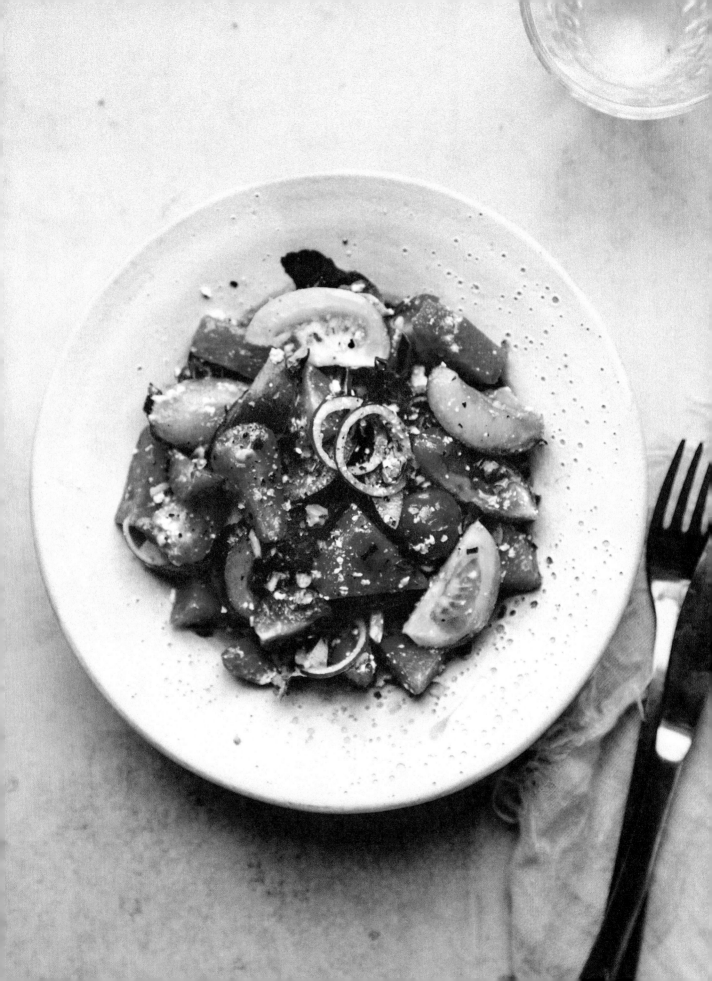

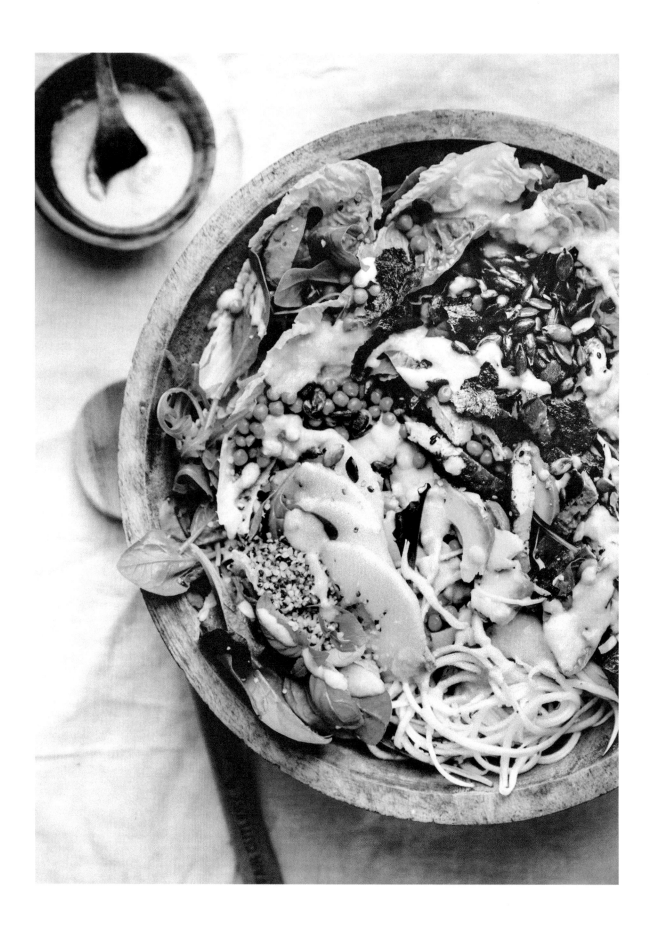

Smoked Tofu and Green Pea Salad

A FAUX FISH SALAD WITH HORSERADISH CREAM

There's a strong tradition of eating smoked fish in northern Europe. However, since I've cut down on fish in a bid to become more environmentally friendly, I'm eating one of my favorite dishes much less—a smoked fish salad that is a specialty in Dutch coastal areas. Happily, I've found a way to make a faux fish salad using smoked tofu and seaweed. This salad is a knockout with a distinct Nordic tang that carries hints of the sea. I've added horseradish, a flavor that's been used for centuries in northern Europe, to deliver a punch that is delicious with the tofu.

Toss the spinach, cabbage, lettuce, and arugula in a large bowl. Add the apple, avocado, zucchini, and peas.

Heat a small skillet over medium-low heat. Add a little of the oil and toast the pumpkin seeds and nori flakes for 2 minutes, stirring to make sure they don't stick. Sprinkle with salt, remove from the pan, and set aside.

Mix the horseradish cream ingredients in a small bowl. Combine in a blender or work it to a smooth consistency with a fork, then set aside.

Return the skillet to medium heat and add a little oil. Cook the tofu cubes with the sesame seeds and ground pepper, stirring constantly, for 2 to 3 minutes. Remove from heat and drizzle with sesame oil and soy sauce.

Add the tofu, pumpkin seeds, and nori flakes to the salad bowl. Top with the hemp seeds. Drizzle with lemon juice and sprinkle with salt. Serve with the horseradish cream.

VE *Use vegan crème fraîche.*
GF *Use gluten-free tamari instead of soy sauce.*

WHY SEAWEED CAN BE THE SOLUTION!
Eating fish today is a complicated issue. Because of intensive fishing in our seas, one of the more urgent environmental crises is happening in our marine ecology. Valuable nutrition like omega-3 fatty acids that we absorb from eating fish originate from what many fish eat—seaweed. Choosing edible seaweed instead can help restore the balance in the seas.

SERVES 2 TO 3
1/4 lb. spinach
1/4 lb. white cabbage leaves, finely shredded
1 head romaine lettuce, leaves separated
2 handfuls of arugula
1 apple, quartered, cored, and sliced
2 avocados, pitted, peeled, and sliced
1 zucchini, spiralized
1/4 lb. green peas, fresh or frozen (defrost at room temperature for 15 minutes)
1 tablespoon canola oil
2 handfuls of pumpkin seeds
1 sheet nori, torn or cut into smaller flakes
7 oz. smoked firm tofu, cut into small cubes
sesame seeds
pinch of ground black pepper
1 tablespoon toasted sesame oil
soy sauce
handful of hemp seeds
juice of 1 lemon
pinch of salt

HORSERADISH CREAM
3/4 cup vegan crème fraîche (see page 50) or dairy crème fraîche
3/4 tablespoon horseradish (or 1 tablespoon wasabi or 1 tablespoon Dijon mustard)
good pinch of salt

Pear and Spicy Seitan Salad

ASIAN PEAR SLAW AND CRISPY SEITAN

This salad combines the fresh tangy flavors of Asian rice rolls (without the fuss of rice papers), with spicy barbecue-style seitan. The addition of pear adds a lovely sweet taste amid the zesty lime and savory flavors. Seitan is one of my favorite meat alternatives. It's not one of the new fabricated mock meats but an ancient food that originated with Buddhist monks who developed alternatives to tofu in the seventh century.

Seitan is made by kneading out the starch from wheat flour and simmering it in broth or soy sauce. It's high in gluten, though, so not an option for those allergic to gluten, who can use jackfruit instead. This fleshy tropical fruit has a texture similar to meat, and a mild taste that acts as a perfect foil to other flavors. You may also substitute firm tofu for the seitan.

Make a marinade by mixing the garlic, lime juice, palm sugar, Sriracha, and soy sauce in a bowl. Drain the seitan well and rub in the marinade.

Heat a skillet over medium-high heat. Add the coconut oil and fry the seitan until crisp.

Arrange the julienned pears, carrots, kohlrabi, and scallions in a bowl, then add the seitan.

Make the lime and soy dressing by mixing all the ingredients. Divide the slaw and seitan between serving bowls, top with avocado and toasted sesame seeds, and drizzle with the dressing.

VE ✓

GF *Use canned jackfruit instead of the seitan. Use gluten-free tamari instead of soy sauce.*

SERVES 4

2 garlic cloves, finely chopped
juice of 1 lime
2 tablespoons palm sugar
1 tablespoon Sriracha or gochugaru (Korean red pepper flakes)
3 tablespoons soy sauce
1 lb. seitan (or use canned green jackfruit or firm tofu)
1–2 tablespoons coconut oil

SLAW

2 Asian or other firm pears, peeled, cored, and julienned (plus extra pears if you'd like to decorate with half a pear per serving)
2 carrots, julienned
1 kohlrabi, peeled and julienned
5 scallions, thinly sliced

LIME AND SOY DRESSING

2 tablespoons soy sauce
juice of 1 lime
1 tablespoon agave syrup
1 teaspoon freshly grated ginger
pinch of gochugaru or other red pepper flakes
1 teaspoon toasted sesame oil
$1\frac{1}{3}$ tablespoons water

2 avocados, pitted, peeled, and sliced
handful of toasted sesame seeds

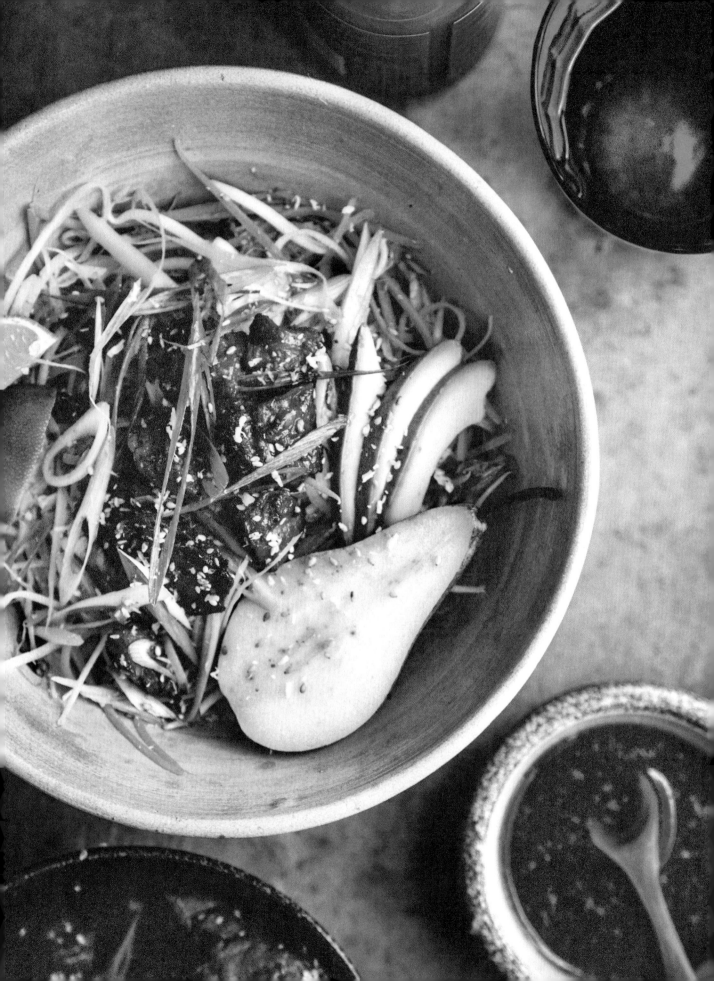

Fig, Pear, and Walnut Salad

SWEET FRUIT, WALNUT, AND GOAT CHEESE WITH CROUTONS

If you visit the south of France in the summer you will most likely find a fresh goat cheese salad on every restaurant menu. Provençal flavors, influenced by both Italian and French cooking, master the fine balance between fresh, sweet, and savory like no other European cuisine. This salad's simple beauty lies in the quality and freshness of the ingredients. It can easily be made with soft vegan nut cheese (see page 155)—or rawmesan (see page 53).

Mix the dressing ingredients, adding enough water to achieve the desired consistency. Taste and adjust with salt and pepper.

Toss all the salad ingredients in a bowl and serve with the dressing.

VE *Substitute vegan cheese (see page 155) for the goat cheese.*

GF *Use gluten-free croutons.*

SERVES 6
6 figs, quartered
1 firm pear, halved, cored, and thinly sliced
1 cup walnuts
8 oz. soft goat cheese, sliced, or chèvre balls (see page 155)
4 avocados, pitted, peeled, and sliced
bunch of mint leaves, chopped
bunch of mixed green leaves (like spinach and arugula)
2 cups sourdough croutons
$1/2$ teaspoon salt

DRESSING
1 garlic clove, finely chopped to a paste
1 shallot, finely diced
4 teaspoons balsamic vinegar
2 tablespoons red wine vinegar
juice of 1 lemon
2 tablespoons tahini
$1/4$ cup extra-virgin olive oil
salt and pepper

BUYING GOOD CHEESE! *When shopping for dairy products it's a good idea to buy organic. Look for products from animals that are grass-fed. Producers who raise grass-fed animals tend to treat their animals better and the products are more often free of contamination from GMOs, pesticides, antibiotics, and growth hormones. Support the farmers and shops who promote a more conscious dairy production. Choosing organic and grass-fed is an investment in better flavor, health, and ecological harmony.*

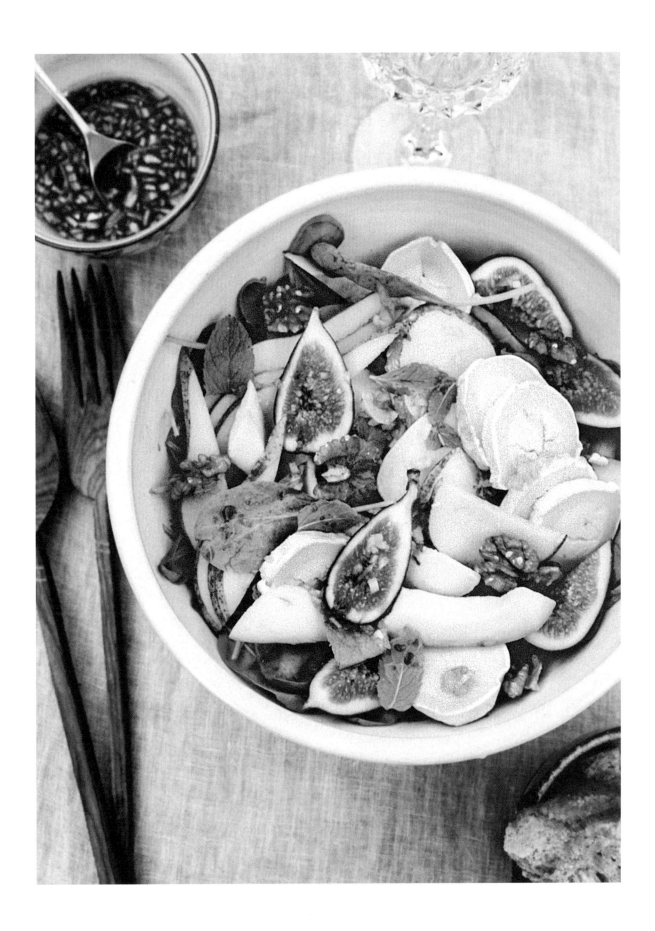

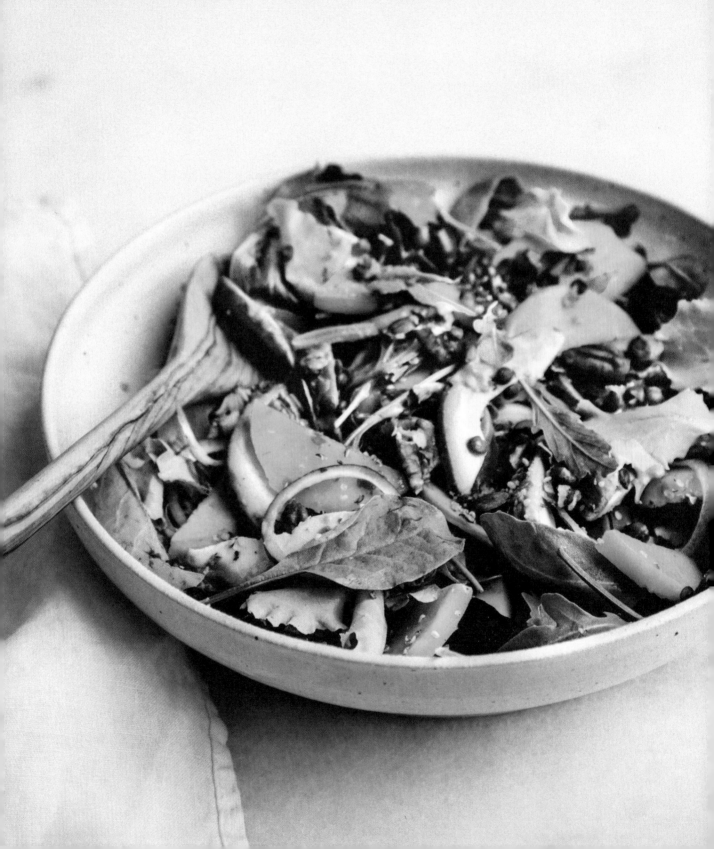

Butternut Squash and Avocado Salad

ROASTED SQUASH, LE PUY LENTILS, AND SOY TAHINI DRESSING

This salad layers avocado, spinach, and walnuts with roasted squash. Together with a savory soy and tahini dressing, it's pure salad perfection.

Preheat the oven to 375°F and line a baking sheet with parchment.

Mix the dressing ingredients, adding enough water to get the consistency right, then set aside.

Halve the butternut squash, scoop out the seeds and fibers, then peel or cut off the skin. Slice each half into slices ¼- to ½-inch thick and cut each slice into smaller, even pieces. Spread out in a single layer on the lined baking sheet. Sprinkle with salt and sage, drizzle with olive oil, and roast for 25 to 30 minutes. Keep an eye on the squash and turn the pieces after about 12 minutes. Remove from the oven when the squash is soft and tender and let cool for 10 to 15 minutes.

Put the salad ingredients and the roasted squash into a bowl. Drizzle with a little extra-virgin olive oil and season with salt and pepper. Divide the salad between four bowls and serve with a good drizzle of soy and tahini dressing.

VE ✓

GF *Use gluten-free tamari instead of soy sauce.*

SERVES 4

1 butternut squash
3 tablespoons freshly chopped sage leaves
olive oil
salt
2 avocados, pitted, peeled, and sliced
1 red onion, sliced into thin rounds
½ cup walnuts, crushed
4–5 cups cooked Le Puy lentils
¼ lb. baby spinach
extra-virgin olive oil
salt and pepper

SOY AND TAHINI DRESSING

¼ cup extra-virgin olive oil
3 tablespoons tamari soy sauce
2 tablespoons tahini paste
¼ cup Japanese rice vinegar
1 garlic clove, finely chopped to a paste
1 tablespoon maple or agave syrup
juice of ½ lemon

OPEN SESAME! *Tahini is literally a wonder product, adding deep flavor whenever it's used. It's a Middle Eastern food staple made from ground sesame seeds and is a key ingredient in hummus (see pages 93 and 156). It also adds depth of flavor to soups, stews, sauces, and baked goods. Tahini can be bought hulled or unhulled. Choose the unhulled variety to enjoy its full nutritional benefits: protein, vitamins, good unsaturated fats, calcium, iron, magnesium, and potassium.*

Apricot and Mozzarella Salad

GRILLED ASPARAGUS, APRICOT, AND MOZZARELLA SALAD WITH SOY DRESSING

There is something so seductive and lush about using fresh stone fruits in salads. Fresh apricots are sun-kissed little wonders that add both sweetness and freshness to this salad. Pairing grilled apricots with mozzarella is an interesting twist on the classic Caprese salad of tomatoes, basil, and mozzarella.

Blend the ingredients for the creamy soy dressing. Taste and adjust the seasoning with salt, then set aside. Put the apricots in a bowl with the asparagus spears and a drizzle of olive oil. Season with salt and pepper and set aside.

Layer the herbs, green leaves, and micro sprouts in a bowl and salt lightly. Gently layer the mozzarella and avocado into the salad.

Preheat a grill or grill pan and cook the asparagus over high heat for 2 to 3 minutes, turning to cook on all sides. Add the asparagus to the salad. Grill the apricots for 2 minutes. Top the salad with the grilled apricots, hemp seeds, and crushed toasted almonds. Serve sprinkled with salt and drizzled with dressing.

VE *Replace mozzarella with a soft vegan cheese. Use agave syrup instead of honey.*

GF ✓

SERVES 2 TO 3

7–8 apricots, pitted and quartered
2 handfuls of baby asparagus
extra-virgin olive oil
3 handfuls of fresh herbs (mint, basil, chives)
bunch of mixed green leaves (I used spinach and arugula)
2 handfuls of fresh and pretty micro sprouts, like red cabbage sprouts, Swiss chard sprouts, radish sprouts, or alfalfa sprouts
5 oz. mozzarella pearls
2 avocados, pitted, peeled, and cut into chunks
salt and pepper

CREAMY SOY DRESSING

3 tablespoons rice vinegar
juice of $1/2$ lemon
1 tablespoon sesame oil
1 tablespoon tamari soy sauce
1 tablespoon honey or agave syrup
1 garlic clove, finely chopped to a paste
1 tablespoon freshly grated ginger
2 tablespoons almond butter
pinch of red pepper flakes
salt

TO SERVE

1 tablespoon hemp seeds
handful of toasted almonds, crushed

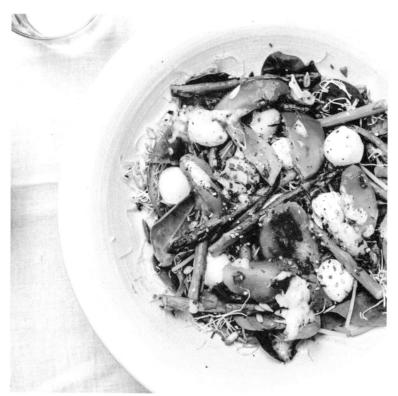

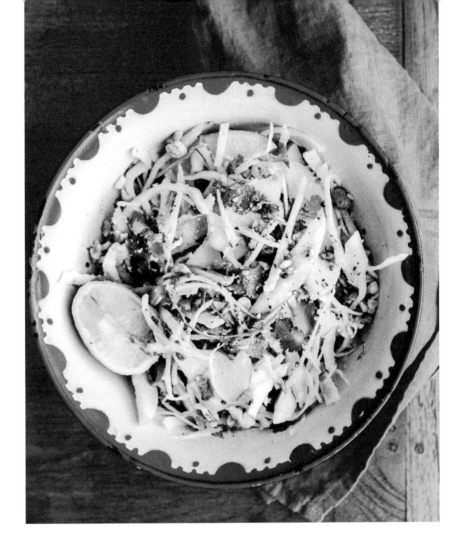

Asian Coleslaw

CILANTRO, LIME, AND PEANUT COLESLAW

Coleslaw delivers a great crunch and balances sweet and savory perfectly. It's a regular on the dinner table in our home and is often varied to fit the rest of the dinner. This Asian-style coleslaw is best served as a cool and refreshing companion to noodles.

Finely shred the cabbage and apple. Mix the coleslaw dressing until smooth, pour over the cabbage, and mix well. Add the cilantro leaves and toasted peanuts. Season with salt and pepper to taste.

VE *Use Vegenaise instead of mayonnaise.*
GF *Use gluten-free tamari instead of soy sauce.*

SERVES 4 AS A SIDE DISH
½ head white cabbage
1 apple, peeled and cored

COLESLAW DRESSING
1 tablespoon peanut butter
1 tablespoon mayonnaise
juice of 1 lime
2 tablespoons rice vinegar
1 garlic clove, crushed
2 tablespoons shoyu soy sauce
1 tablespoon toasted sesame oil
2 tablespoons extra-virgin olive oil

2 handfuls of cilantro leaves
2 handfuls of toasted peanuts
salt and pepper

Midsummer Salad

HERBED BABY POTATOES WITH EGGS, YOGURT, AND MUSTARD

Midsummer is without a doubt my favorite Swedish holiday. We eat alfresco, wear flowers in our hair, and dance barefoot with our children. The Midsummer table is usually a buffet of rustic Scandinavian dishes and there are always plenty of freshly picked new potatoes to enjoy. This festive bowl brings you the essential Nordic Midsummer flavors, with new potato salad, eggs, and fresh herbs.

Boil the eggs for 6 to 7 minutes, rinse under cold running water, and set aside. Cook the new potatoes for 15 minutes in plenty of water with a good pinch of salt and a few dill stalks. You don't need to peel baby potatoes, just scrub them before cooking if they need it. Drain the potatoes, drizzle with olive oil, sprinkle with salt, and set aside to cool.

Mix the ingredients for the dressing, adding water to achieve the desired consistency. Taste and adjust the seasoning with salt and set aside. Cut the potatoes into bite-size pieces and place with the rest of the salad ingredients in a big bowl. Give it a grind of salt and pepper and drizzle with the dressing. Toss gently to coat everything in dressing. Peel and halve the eggs and serve with the salad and, as we say in Swedish, *Njut av maten!*—Enjoy the meal!

VE *Use vegan crème fraîche or other vegan alternative for the sour cream. Use Vegenaise instead of mayonnaise. Omit the eggs.*

GF ✓

SERVES 4

4 medium eggs
2 lbs. baby new potatoes
2 bunches of fresh dill, fronds roughly chopped, stalks reserved for cooking the potatoes
extra-virgin olive oil
1 red onion, thinly sliced
handful of chives, roughly chopped
¼ lb. mixed green leaves (I used baby spinach or arugula)
1 sweet apple (I used pink lady), quartered, cored, and thinly sliced
½ cucumber, sliced
small handful of capers
salt and pepper

MUSTARD DRESSING
⅓ cup yogurt or sour cream
⅓ cup mayonnaise
juice of 1 lemon
1 tablespoon apple cider vinegar
1 tablespoon Dijon mustard

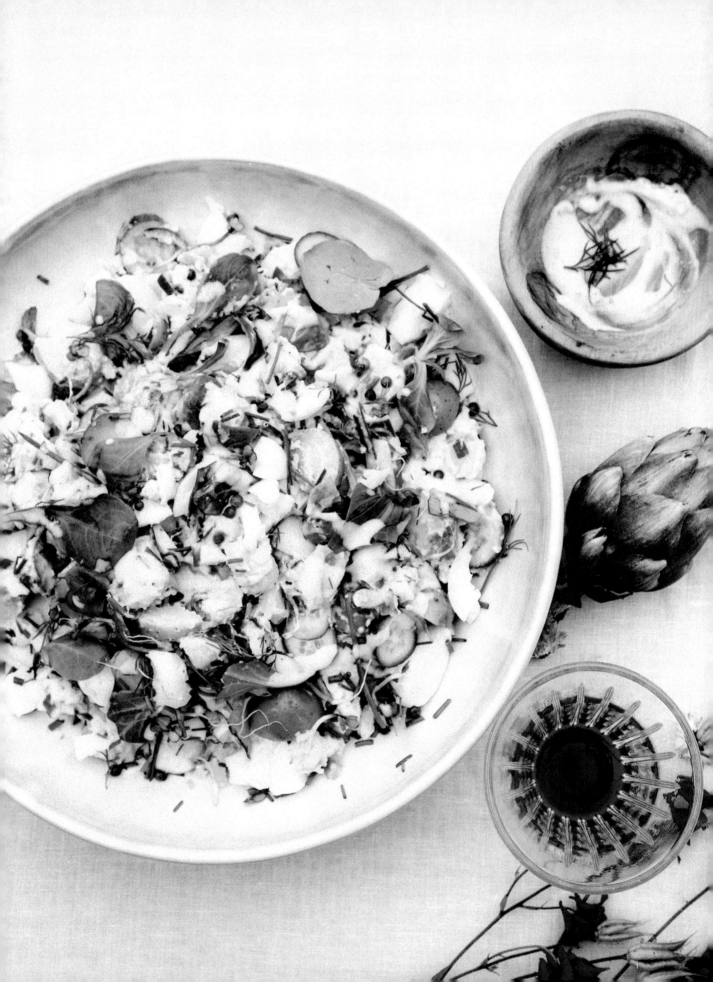

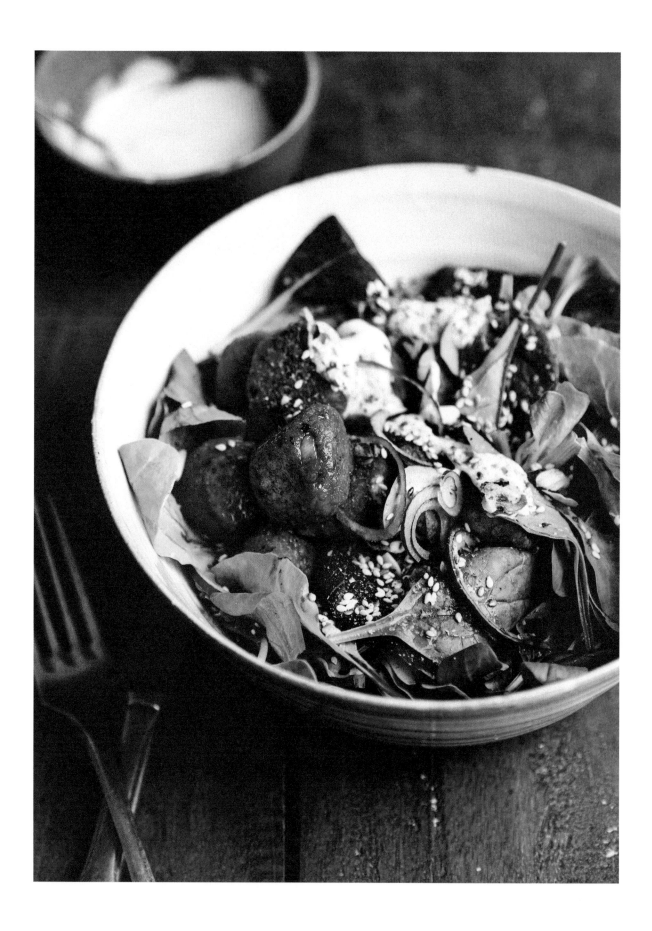

Beet Falafel, Dukkah, and Mint Salad

BEET FALAFEL WITH DUKKAH, MINT SALAD, AND YOGURT

These beet and chickpea falafels have more to offer than meets the eye. They're boosted with extra heat from spicy harissa and make a perfect partner for a salad of fresh greens and cool mint. Middle Eastern salads are everything but bland—always simple and to the point. The falafels are pan-fried, not deep-fried, for a fresher, lighter taste. Chickpeas, which are the main ingredient in falafel, are a superb source of plant-based protein.

Roughly process the dukkah ingredients in a food processor and set aside.

Wipe out the food processor and add the falafel ingredients. Process carefully, just pulsing a few times, without overblending (you want to see pieces left in the mix). Roll small balls with your hands and refrigerate them for 20 to 30 minutes.

Mix the chopped mint and parsley with the green leaves and onion. Drizzle with lemon juice and olive oil and sprinkle with salt and pepper to taste. Heat a skillet over medium-high heat and add a drizzle of olive oil. Cook the beet falafels on all sides. Divide the mint salad between serving bowls. Add the beet falafel and serve with yogurt and sprinkles of dukkah.

VE *Substitute vegan yogurt or vegan crème*
fraiche (see page 50) for the Greek yogurt.
GF ✓

INISO THE BEAT *Beets make a great natural food coloring and provide excellent health benefits. They're especially valuable in aiding our liver functions, helping the body's cleansing system to work at its best. It's a good idea to use the beet leaves if you have a fresh bunch as the leaves are exceptionally nutritious and can be used in place of spinach and lettuce.*

SERVES 2 AS A MAIN COURSE
OR 3 AS A STARTER

DUKKAH
1/4 cup mixed nuts, such as
   pistachio and almonds
1 1/2 tablespoons sesame seeds
1 1/2 tablespoons ground coriander
2 teaspoons ground cumin
1/2 teaspoon sea salt
a good pinch of red pepper flakes

BEET FALAFELS
   (makes 15 small falafels)
1 small raw beet, finely grated
2 medium carrots, grated
2 shallots, diced
1 teaspoon ground coriander
14 1/2 oz. can chickpeas, drained
1 tablespoon harissa paste
1/2 tablespoon ground cumin
2 garlic cloves
1 1/2 cups chickpea flour
1 teaspoon salt

MINT SALAD
1 handful of mint leaves, roughly
   chopped
1 handful of flat-leaf parsley,
   roughly chopped
8 oz. mixed green leaves—use
   interesting ones like mesclun
   or arugula
1 red onion, finely sliced
juice of 1 lemon
extra-virgin olive oil
salt and pepper

TO SERVE
1/2 cup Greek yogurt

Moroccan Harissa Salad

SPICY HARISSA CAULIFLOWER WITH CARROT AND ORANGE TAHINI DRESSING

This North African salad is a pure flavor party that marries spicy harissa-marinated cauliflower with powerful tahini, softened by cool and creamy avocado and sweet carrot. To make this salad unforgettable, drizzle with the orange-flavored dressing and top with almonds.

Preheat the oven to 400°F and line a baking sheet with parchment.

Blend the dressing ingredients into a smooth sauce, adding small amounts of water while blending until it is at your desired consistency. Store in the fridge until ready to serve.

Arrange the cauliflower on the lined baking sheet. Mix the olive oil with the harissa and pour over the cauliflower, making sure they are well coated. Sprinkle with salt and roast with the red onion wedges for 35 to 40 minutes. Toss cauliflower and onion wedges after 20 minutes. Once tender, remove from the oven.

Mix the roasted veggies with the carrot, avocado, raisins, and almonds. Top with sesame seeds and mint leaves. Serve with the tahini dressing.

VE ✓ GF ✓

SERVES 4

2 tablespoons olive oil
1/4 cup harissa Mina sauce (or
    2 tablespoons harissa paste with
    2 tablespoons water)
1 medium cauliflower, florets
    separated
salt
2 red onions, cut in wedges
8 carrots, shaved into thin bands
4 avocados, pitted, peeled, and
    cut into small pieces
1/2 cup raisins
3/4 cup toasted almonds

ORANGE TAHINI DRESSING
juice and zest of 1 orange
1 garlic clove
3/4 teaspoon salt
1/4 cup tahini
2 tablespoons agave or maple syrup
2 tablespoons extra-virgin olive oil

TO SERVE
sesame seeds
Moroccan mint leaves

HARISSA! *Harissa is a delicious chile pepper paste used in North African and Middle Eastern kitchens. The recipe varies from home to home and between regions, and many home cooks have a personal tweak or secret ingredient. A quality harissa takes time and love to prepare—slowly cooking onions, bell peppers, and chile peppers with spices to release sweet and deep flavors. An absolute favorite of mine is a sauce from Mina (www.casablancafoods.com), that's vegan and additive free, with a delicious home-cooked taste. Mina harissa is available in many supermarkets or easy to order from their website or on Amazon. One tablespoon of harissa paste is equivalent to 2 tablespoons Mina harissa sauce.*

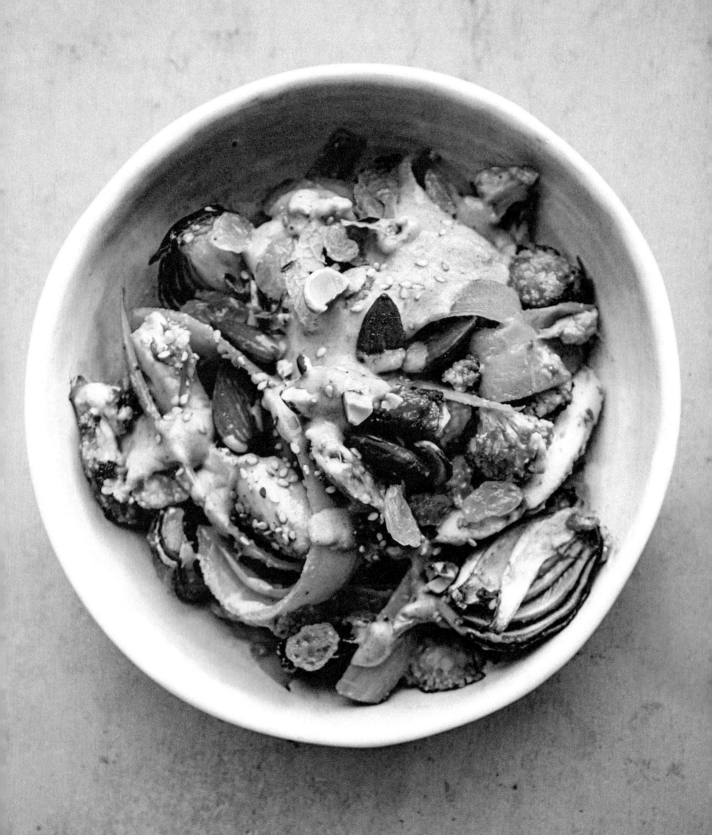

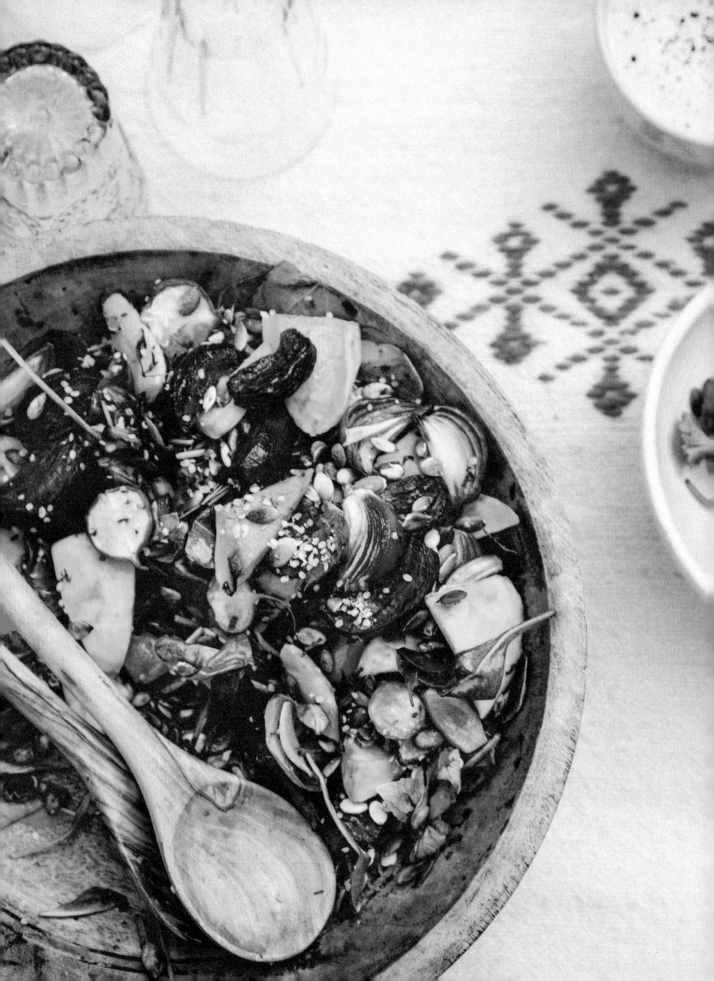

Pumpkin Salad

ROASTED PUMPKIN, BEET, AND CRISPY HERBS WITH LEMON TAHINI DRESSING

This colorful pumpkin salad is a feast for all senses and adding herbs while roasting creates delicious aromas as well as flavor. It's a filling salad that even dedicated meat lovers like, and makes a great buffet dish. The tangy tahini dressing brightens up the intense flavor of the roasted vegetables and herbs.

Preheat the oven to 400°F and line two baking sheets with parchment. Mix the dressing ingredients, slowly adding enough water until it is the desired consistency, then set aside.

Scoop out the pumpkin seeds and fibers, then peel or cut off the skin. Cut the flesh into bite-size wedges.

To toast the pumpkin seeds, first rinse them in a sieve under running water. Place them in a saucepan and cover generously with water. Bring to a boil and let the seeds simmer for 10 minutes, then drain. Transfer them to one of the baking sheets, sprinkle with a pinch of salt and roast until golden and fragrant, about 5 minutes, checking frequently to make sure they don't burn.

Peel and cut the beets and onions into bite-size wedges and halve the radishes. Spread the beets, onions, and pumpkin in a single layer on the second baking sheet. Drizzle with olive oil and sprinkle with salt, thyme, sage, and tarragon. Roast for about 25 minutes, turning halfway through, until the pumpkin and beets are softened. Keep an eye on the oven during the last 5 minutes so they don't overcook.

Place the roasted veggies and radishes in a bowl and toss with the spinach and toasted seeds. Serve with the tahini dressing.

VE ✓ GF ✓

SERVES 4

½ a small pumpkin (about ¾ lb.)
¾ lb. beets (about 8 medium)
2 red onions
bunch of radishes
olive oil
salt
handful of fresh thyme
small handful of sage, chopped
small handful of tarragon
bunch of baby spinach
handful of hemp seeds

LEMON TAHINI DRESSING

2 tablespoons tahini
juice of ½ lemon
1 garlic clove, finely chopped
   to a paste
3 tablespoons extra-virgin olive oil
1 teaspoon maple syrup
salt and pepper

SEEDS OF JOY! *Feeling tense? Three-quarters cup of pumpkin seeds almost covers the daily requirement of magnesium that helps our muscles and bodies relax. They also contain compounds that boost our mood and can be efficient in fighting depression. The seeds are full of fiber and protein and are great for keeping your weight in check. Roast them to break down phytic acids and to release the maximum flavor.*

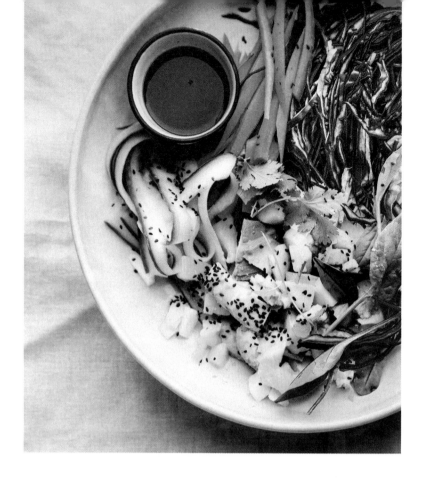

CHOOSING SOY! *Soy sauce is a great Asian flavor. If made by the traditional fermentation process, it's a healthy ingredient. Stay clear of the chemical soy sauces that are made without full fermentation as they often contain harmful substances due to the rapid processing of the soybeans. A tip is to look for Japanese soy—shoyu or tamari soy sauce—rather than Chinese soy. Whole food shops usually stock the best soy sauces.*

Spring Thai Salad

RAW SALAD WITH MANGO, CILANTRO, AND LIME SOY DRESSING

This invigorating, mainly raw, salad has a fresh lightness. The soy dressing adds a contrast to the sweetness of the mango and makes this salad full flavored.

Mix the ingredients for the soy dressing.

Slice the scallions in fine rounds and shred the red cabbage. Halve, pit, peel, and cut the mango and avocado into small dice. Shave the cucumber into thin bands and cut the carrots into sticks.

Divide the cut salad ingredients into bowls and add the cilantro and spinach. Sprinkle with sesame seeds and serve with the dressing on the side.

Tip! For a bigger meal, add quinoa, smoked tofu, and cashews.

VE ✓
GF *Use gluten-free tamari instead of soy sauce.*

SERVES 2 TO 3
3 scallions
¼ small red cabbage
1 mango
2 avocados
½ cucumber
3 carrots
big handful of cilantro leaves
2–3 handfuls of baby spinach
toasted sesame seeds
¾ cup cooked quinoa (optional)
8 oz. smoked tofu, diced (optional)
½ cup toasted cashews (optional)

LIME SOY DRESSING
½ cup soy sauce
juice of 2 limes
3 tablespoons coconut sugar
½ teaspoon freshly grated ginger
2 tablespoons water
1 tablespoon toasted sesame oil

Kale Caesar

KALE, AVOCADO, AND ROMAINE CAESAR WITH HEMP AND WALNUT PARM

This salad is my take on one of the world's most famous dishes—Caesar salad. There are plenty of delicious vegan versions out in the ether, proving that there are many roads to Rome or—should we say—to Caesar salad! This recipe has kale as well as romaine lettuce, enhancing its nourishing goodness. Golden sourdough croutons and buttery avocado contrast with the crispy lettuce and zesty Caesar dressing in this salad bowl.

In a blender, mix the dressing ingredients to form a smooth sauce and set aside. Blend the ingredients roughly for the hemp and walnut parm (or grate 2 tablespoons Parmesan if you are not making a vegan version). Tear the sourdough bread into small pieces.

Heat a skillet over medium-high heat and add the olive oil. Toast the bread pieces on all sides, sprinkle with salt, then remove from the heat. Put the kale and romaine lettuce in a bowl and drizzle with ½ cup of the Caesar dressing. Work the dressing into the salad leaves. Slice the avocado into small wedges and add to the bowl with the sourdough croutons. Sprinkle with the Parmesan or hemp and walnut parm.

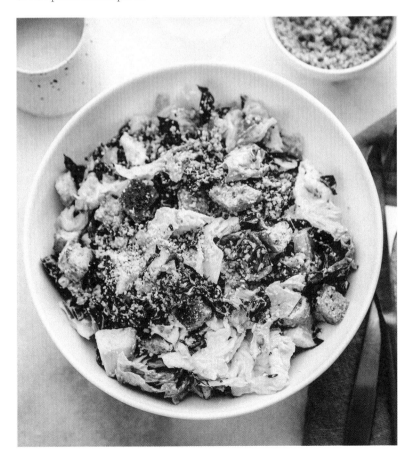

SERVES 4
2–3 slices sourdough bread
1 tablespoon olive oil
salt
½ lb. curly baby kale
8 romaine lettuce leaves, torn into pieces
4 avocados, pitted and peeled

CAESAR DRESSING
(makes about 1 cup)
⅔ cup raw cashews, soaked for at least 4 hours
½ cup water
juice of ½ lemon
1 teaspoon Dijon mustard
1 teaspoon capers (optional)
2 garlic cloves, sliced
2 tablespoons finely grated Parmesan
1 teaspoon salt
¼ cup extra-virgin olive oil

HEMP AND WALNUT PARM
(can be used in place of Parmesan)
½ cup hemp seeds
½ cup walnuts
2 tablespoon nutritional yeast
pinch of salt

VE *Use nutritional yeast or the walnut hemp parm instead of Parmesan.*
GF ✓

KALE YEAH! *Kale is one of the healthiest foods you can eat. It has anti-inflammatory, cholesterol-lowering properties that are linked to reducing the risks of serious diseases.*

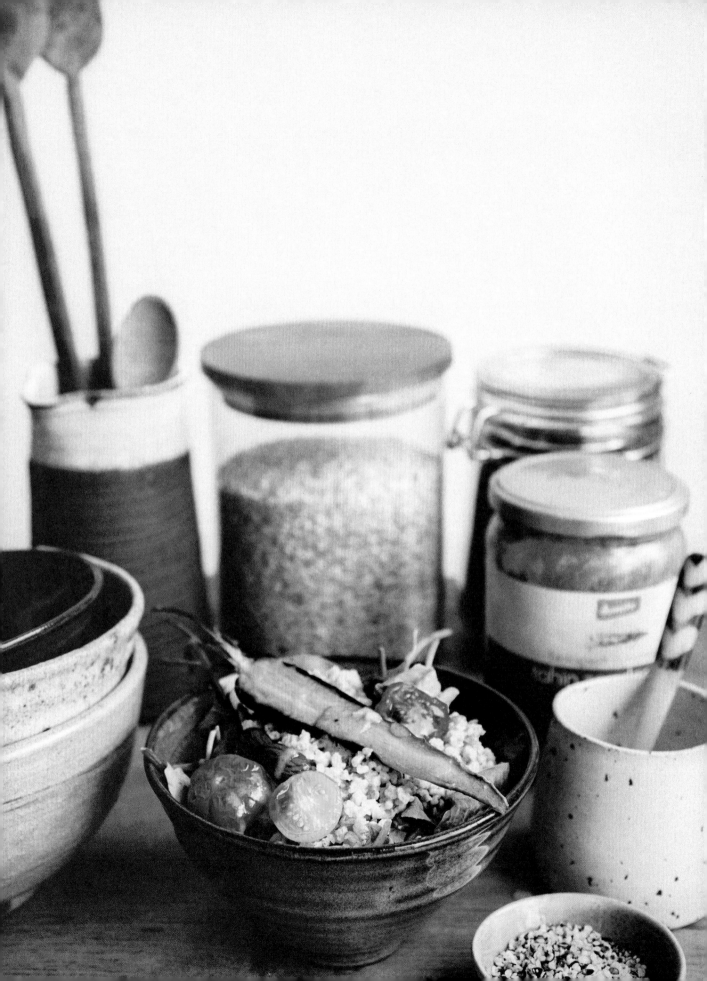

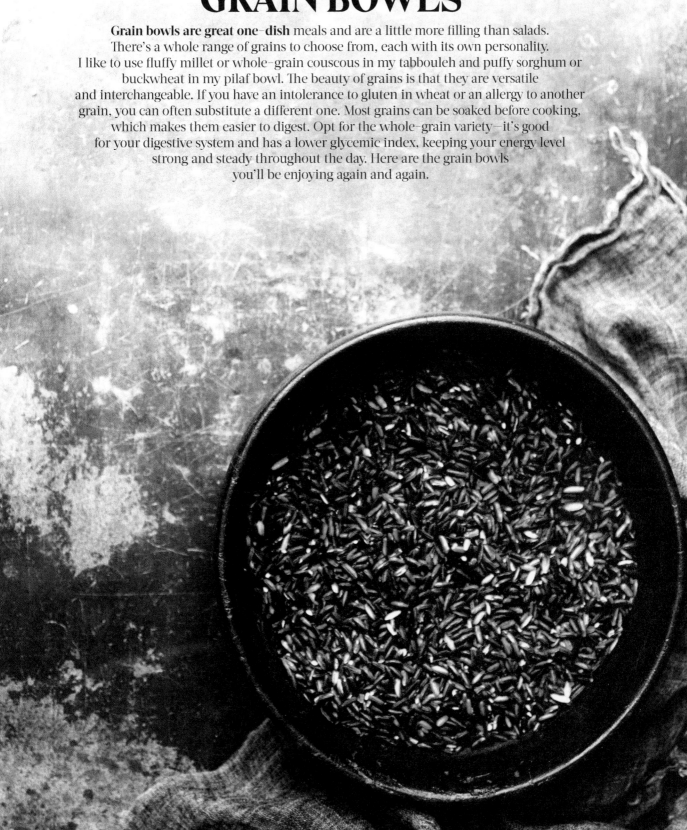

GRAIN BOWLS

Grain bowls are great one-dish meals and are a little more filling than salads.
There's a whole range of grains to choose from, each with its own personality.
I like to use fluffy millet or whole-grain couscous in my tabbouleh and puffy sorghum or
buckwheat in my pilaf bowl. The beauty of grains is that they are versatile
and interchangeable. If you have an intolerance to gluten in wheat or an allergy to another
grain, you can often substitute a different one. Most grains can be soaked before cooking,
which makes them easier to digest. Opt for the whole-grain variety—it's good
for your digestive system and has a lower glycemic index, keeping your energy level
strong and steady throughout the day. Here are the grain bowls
you'll be enjoying again and again.

Rainbow Grain Bowl

BUCKWHEAT, BEAN SPROUTS, VEGETABLES, AND FRUIT WITH GREEN GODDESS DRESSING

A rainbow grain bowl! Don't you just love the color explosion here? The idea is to gather vegetables and fruit of different colors in groups for a rainbow effect. Expect to be flexible when choosing ingredients for a rainbow grain bowl—go with your most vibrant market finds. Food of similar colors often share the same nutrients, meaning a rainbow meal provides a variety of goodness.

Bring out the flavor of each ingredient by steaming or roasting. Or just work with raw cut vegetables.

The addition of grains upgrades your grain bowl to a more filling meal. Buckwheat is perfect, deliciously puffy and bouncy! Toast it before cooking for an extra nutty flavor. I bind it all together with a flavorful green goddess dressing made with creamy avocado and herbs.

Preheat the oven to 400°F. Line a baking sheet with parchment and roast any suitable vegetables, such as radishes and tomatoes, for 20 minutes.

Make the dressing by combining the ingredients in a food processor and blending until smooth, adding water until you reach your desired consistency.

Heat a saucepan with a drizzle of olive oil and toast the buckwheat, stirring constantly, for 2 minutes. Cover with water and add a pinch of salt, then bring to a boil. Let the buckwheat simmer for 10 minutes, or until tender, then drain and spread it out on a clean dishtowel to dry for 10 minutes.

Steam or boil the cauliflower and broccoli for 4 minutes. Rinse under cold water, drain, and set aside.

Divide the buckwheat between four serving bowls and add the rest of the ingredients either in groups by color or mixed together. Season with salt and pepper to taste. Serve with the green goddess dressing.

Tip! Make this a super bowl by adding chickpeas or beans for extra protein.

VE ✓ GF ✓

SERVES 4

bunch of colorful raw vegetables (rainbow or regular carrots, chioggia beets, radishes, and tomatoes), cut in pieces or sliced
olive oil
1 cup buckwheat
handful of cauliflower and broccoli florets
bunch of spinach
1 mango, halved, pitted, peeled, and diced
3 handfuls of shredded red cabbage
2 handfuls of seeds and nuts (I used hemp seeds and toasted almonds)
sprouts (I used bean sprouts and beet sprouts)
handful of strawberries
salt and pepper

GREEN GODDESS DRESSING
1 avocado, pitted and peeled
1 garlic clove
juice of $\frac{1}{2}$ lemon
handful of chopped chives
handful of parsley
$1\frac{1}{2}$ tablespoons fresh tarragon
salt and pepper

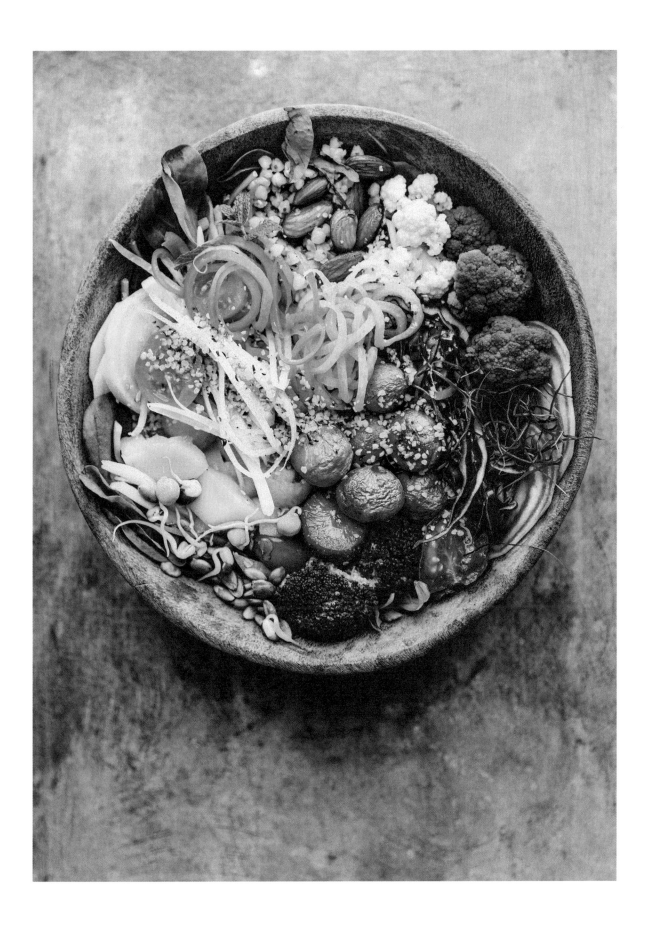

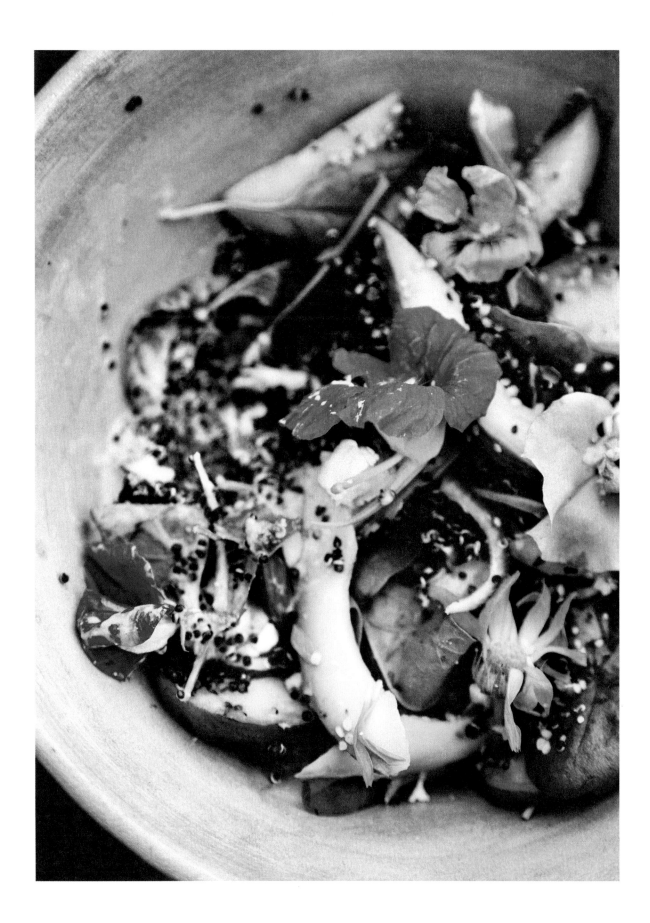

Flower Power

BLACK QUINOA, PEACH, CHÈVRE, FLOWERS, AND ORANGE BLOSSOM DRESSING

This bowl celebrates the beauty of summer. Flowers have subtle flavors, ranging from sweet to peppery, and they fit perfectly in light and fresh salads.

This bowl has a base of crunchy black quinoa cooked in a broth with herbs. Peach and avocado add a sweet and buttery smoothness, while the creamy almond and tahini dressing with orange blossom water adds an interesting finish. This salad is a lovely side dish or festive addition to a buffet.

Pour the broth into a medium saucepan and add the quinoa and thyme. Bring to a boil before lowering the heat, then simmer for 15 minutes. Drain the quinoa and allow to cool.

Mix the dressing ingredients to a smooth sauce and add water slowly until you have your desired consistency.

Divide the salad ingredients, except the flowers and goat cheese, between four serving bowls. Add the lentils if you want a fuller meal. Season with salt and pepper to taste. Top with the edible flowers, goat cheese, and almonds. Serve with the dressing.

Tip! Add cooked lentils to make this a more filling meal.

VE *Use vegan cashew cheese instead of goat cheese (see page 155).*

GF ✓

SERVES 4

2 cups vegetable broth
1 cup black quinoa
2 tablespoons finely chopped thyme
bunch of baby spinach
2–3 peaches, pitted and cut into wedges
2 avocados, pitted, peeled, and sliced
2 handfuls flowers, like nasturtium, marigolds, and viola
8 oz. soft goat cheese, crumbled
2½ cups cooked firm lentils (optional)
2 handfuls of toasted almonds, crushed
salt and pepper

ORANGE BLOSSOM DRESSING

3 tablespoons extra-virgin olive oil
½ teaspoon orange blossom water
2 tablespoons almond butter
½ teaspoon agave syrup
1 tablespoon tahini
juice of ½ lemon
1 garlic clove, finely chopped to a paste
salt and pepper

EDIBLE FLOWERS! *Flowers add lightness and soothing scents to food. Though many flowers are edible, not all are. It's not safe to eat unknown flowers found in the wild as some can be poisonous. You can grow your own or buy them in stores. Popular edible flowers include elderflower, lavender, viola, rose, calendula, dandelion, chive blossoms, and nasturtium.*

Farro and Heirloom Tomatoes

FARRO WITH ROASTED HEIRLOOM TOMATOES, BALSAMIC DRESSING, AND BURRATA

Grains become a lot more interesting if they get a little extra attention. I toast my farro before I cook it, which adds an extra nutty flavor. This method works well with all grains. Farro is a wheat grain similar to spelt and it comes in three varieties—whole-grain, semi-pearled, and pearled. The whole farro grain is the healthiest of the three and the one that takes longest to cook. Pre-soaking it for 8 hours is nutritionally beneficial and it shortens the cooking time.

Preheat the oven to 400°F and line a baking sheet with parchment.

Heat a large saucepan over medium-high heat and toast the farro, stirring constantly, for 4 to 5 minutes. Add 4 cups of water with a good pinch of salt and the rosemary and bring to a boil. Turn down the heat to simmer. Whole-grain pre-soaked farro cooks in 40 minutes. Pre-soaked semi-pearled farro cooks in 20 to 25 minutes, and pearled farro cooks in 15 minutes with no soaking needed.

Taste the farro. It should have a good bite, but not be too mushy. Remove the rosemary and drain the farro well. Spread onto a clean dishtowel and let it dry for 10 to 15 minutes.

Meanwhile, arrange the tomatoes on the lined baking sheet, cut side up, with the onion. Drizzle with olive oil, sprinkle with salt, and roast for 25 minutes.

Whisk the dressing ingredients together and set aside.

In a dry skillet, toast the pine nuts until fragrant.

Rinse and drain the cannellini beans and pat dry with paper towels. Put the beans, farro, roasted tomatoes and onions, olives, and herbs in a bowl and mix well. Drizzle with the balsamic dressing. Taste and adjust the seasoning with salt and pepper. Serve in bowls topped with creamy pieces of burrata and basil leaves.

VE *Replace the burrata with vegan cheese.*

GF *Use buckwheat instead of farro and cook according to the package instructions.*

SERVES 4

1¼ cups farro, preferably whole-grain, pre-soaked for 8 hours
few sprigs of fresh rosemary
¾ lb. heirloom cherry tomatoes of different colors, halved or quartered according to size
2 red onions, quartered
olive oil
2 handfuls of toasted pine nuts
14½ oz. can cannellini beans
¼ lb. black olives, pitted
bunch of mixed fresh herbs, such as purple basil, parsley, and mint, chopped
salt and pepper

BALSAMIC DRESSING

⅓ cup extra-virgin olive oil
juice of 1 lemon
1 garlic clove, finely chopped to a paste
3 tablespoons balsamic vinegar
pinch of salt and pepper

TO SERVE

burrata or vegan mozzarella
basil leaves

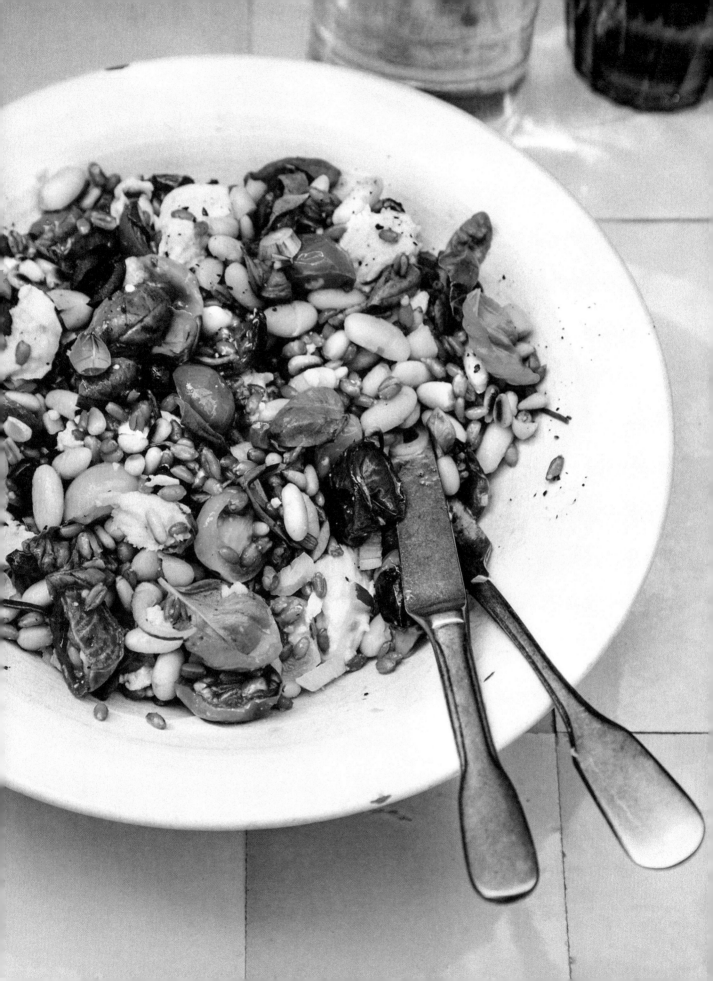

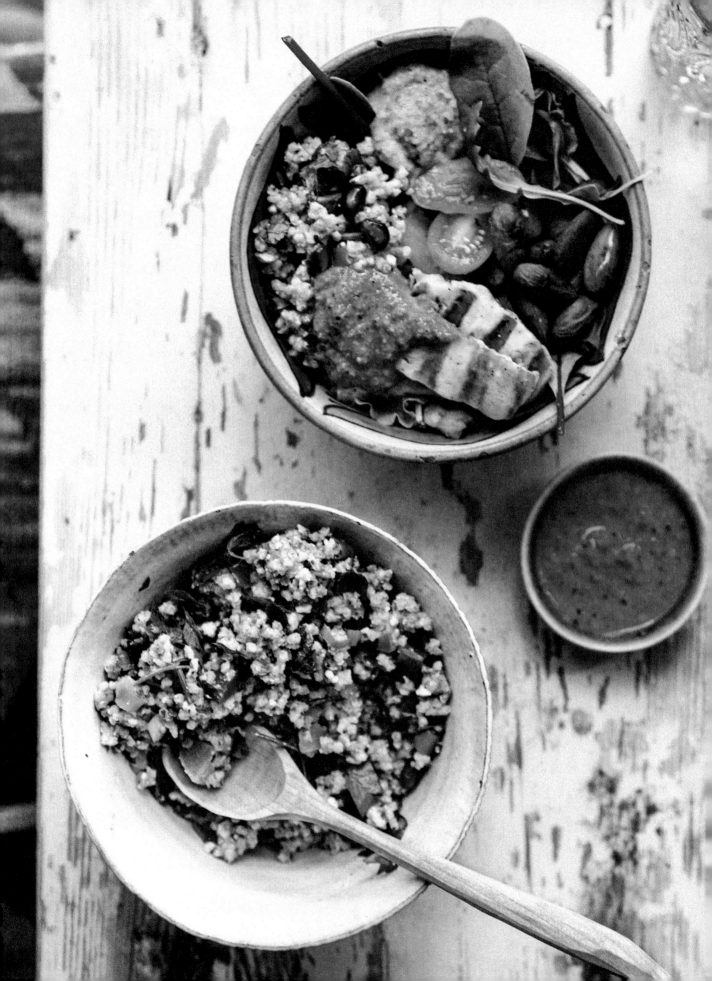

Meze Bowl

GRILLED HALLOUMI WITH TABBOULEH, CILANTRO HUMMUS, AND ALMOND MUHAMMARA

I first discovered the wonders of meze—a sort of Middle Eastern tapas meal, an array of fully flavored snacks, salads, and dipping sauces—in Turkish and Lebanese restaurants while living in one of Europe's most diverse and exciting cities: London. Inspired by chefs like Yotam Ottolenghi I was soon making meze at home.

This bowl mixes flavors of zesty lemon with fresh vegetables and vibrant herbs, using tabbouleh (see page 152) and nutty tahini dips. The grilled halloumi balances the fresh tabbouleh with a salty buttery taste. A meze meal is flexible by nature, so feel free to add your own tweaks. For example, you could swap the halloumi for falafel (see page 77) or roasted chickpeas.

First blend the ingredients for the muhammara in a food processor and set aside. Then blend the hummus ingredients and set aside.

Heat a grill pan and add a small drizzle of olive oil. Fry the halloumi for 2 to 3 minutes on each side.

Serve with the muhammara, hummus, tabbouleh, mesclun, and cherry tomatoes. Top with toasted almonds.

Tip! I've used preserved grilled red peppers in oil for the muhammara because the flavor deepens during preservation, but you can also roast red peppers at 450°F for 35 minutes.

VE *Replace the halloumi with falafel or roasted chickpeas.*

GF *Substitute gluten-free bread for pita bread.*

SERVES 4
olive oil
1 lb. halloumi, sliced
4 cups prepared tabbouleh, (see
    page 152), plain cooked bulgur,
    or other grain
bunch of mesclun or arugula
handful of cherry tomatoes
4 handfuls of toasted almonds

ALMOND MUHAMMARA
1/2 cup grilled red bell peppers,
    in oil
handful toasted almonds or
    walnuts (save some for topping)
2 garlic cloves
1/2 teaspoon Aleppo pepper flakes or
    red pepper flakes of your choice
juice of 1 lemon
salt

CILANTRO HUMMUS
14 1/2 oz. can chickpeas, drained
2 garlic cloves, crushed
3 tablespoons tahini
1/2 teaspoon salt
zest and juice of 1 lime
bunch of cilantro leaves
drizzle of extra-virgin olive oil

SUGGESTED ADDITIONS
olives
yogurt
pita bread

Buddha Bowl

SPICY CHICKPEAS, TOFU, QUINOA, AND SPROUTS WITH TURMERIC DRESSING

Buddha bowls are wholesome dishes so full to the brim that the heap of food resembles the rounded belly of Buddha. I make them to share and hand out individual bowls at the table.

Packed with protein-rich quinoa, chickpeas, and roasted sweet potato—plus turmeric, which is renowned for its health-giving properties—this is an extra-nourishing Buddha bowl. You can easily customize it by adding or substituting similar ingredients.

Cook the quinoa according to the package instructions, then drain and set aside. Blend the ingredients for the turmeric dressing and set aside.

Heat a skillet over medium-high heat and add 1 to 2 tablespoons coconut oil. Cook the sweet potato cubes for a couple of minutes until tender, then remove from the pan. Wipe out the pan and reheat it with 1 to 2 tablespoons coconut oil. Cook the chickpeas for 2 to 3 minutes, then sprinkle with cayenne, ground coriander, and salt. Remove from the heat and set aside.

In a bowl, stir together the soy sauce, ginger, and maple syrup. Wipe out the pan and add the tofu and fry until golden, a couple of minutes. Drizzle with the soy mixture and cook for another minute. Remove from the heat.

Build the Buddha bowl with a base of quinoa and green leaves, then add the chickpeas, tofu, and sweet potato with the rest of the ingredients. Serve with the turmeric dressing.

VE ✓

GF *Use gluten-free tamari instead of soy sauce.*

SERVES 2 TO 3

1 cup quinoa

coconut oil

4 sweet potatoes, peeled and diced

14½ oz. can chickpeas

pinch of cayenne pepper

½ teaspoon ground coriander

2 tablespoons soy sauce

1 teaspoon freshly grated ginger

1 tablespoon maple or agave syrup

¼ lb. firm tofu, pressed (see page 16) and cubed

½ lb. melon, cut into bite-size pieces

bunch of radishes, cleaned

fresh green leaves, such as mesclun or arugula

3 carrots, spiralized

¼ lb. micro sprouts

salt and pepper

TURMERIC DRESSING

¼ cup tahini

2 tablespoons almond or cashew butter

juice of 2 lemons

3 tablespoons olive oil

½ teaspoon freshly grated or ground turmeric

½ teaspoon ground cumin

salt and pepper

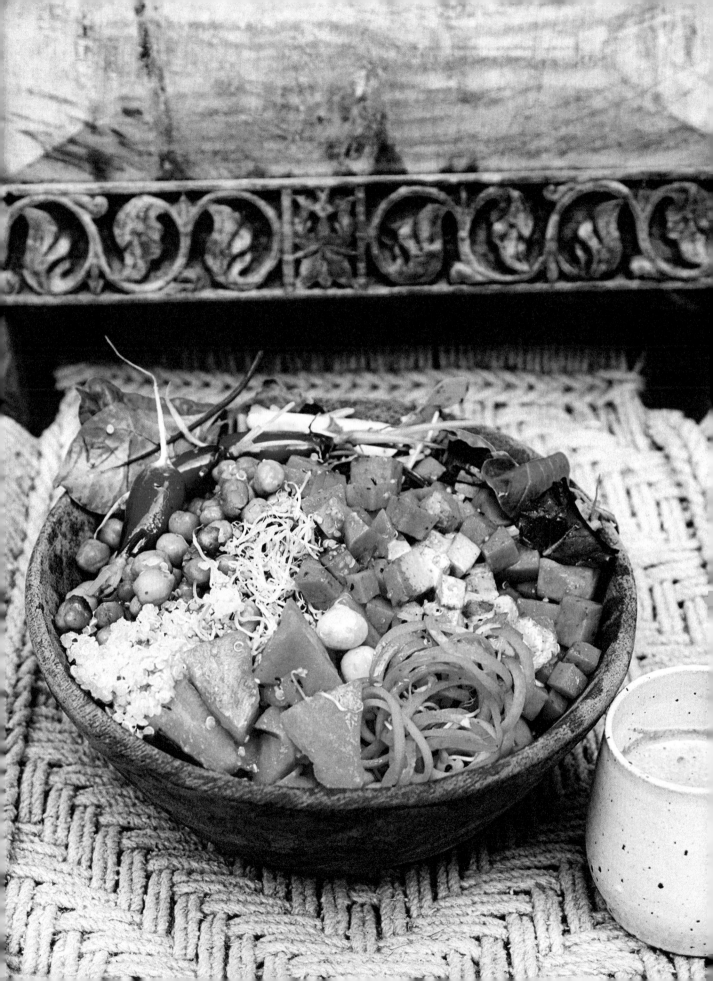

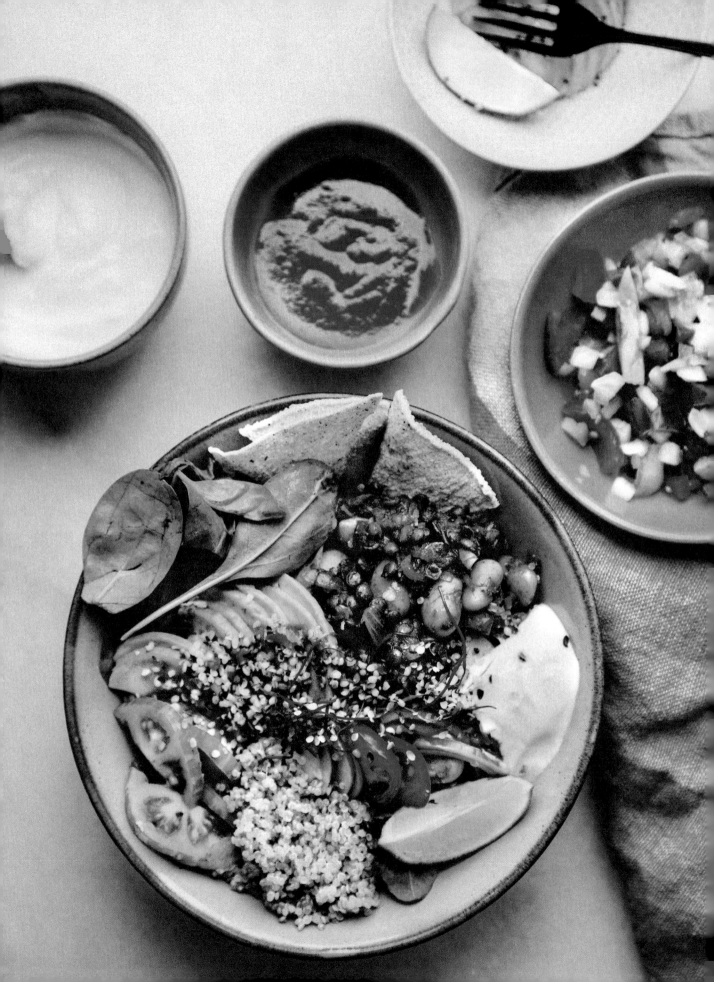

Baja Mexican

SPICY BEANS WITH LIME SAUCE, QUINOA, AND SALSA

Mexican is one of the most popular cuisines in our house, especially when the kids get to choose. The bonus of Mexican taco-style meals is the pick-and-mix flexibility of adding hot sauce and other ingredients to taste. Oregano, cumin, chile powder, and paprika add distinct Mexican flavor to the beans.

You can use any mixture of beans or lentils, or just one. Other signature flavors for a Mexican bowl are salsa and Baja sauce.

Cook the quinoa according to the package instructions, then drain and set aside. Mix the ingredients for the salsa and the Baja sauce and set aside.

Heat a skillet and add a drizzle of olive oil. Cook the shallots over medium-low heat until translucent. Add another drizzle of olive oil and the rest of the spicy bean ingredients, cooking for 5 minutes over low heat.

Divide the quinoa and spicy beans in serving bowls. Add the avocado, lime wedges, tortilla chips, salsa, and Baja sauce. Serve with hot sauce, hemp seeds, and spinach leaves.

Tip! Use avocado instead of the sour cream for making the Baja sauce.

VE *Use vegan crème fraiche, soygurt, or avocado instead of sour cream.*
GF ✓

NOT ALL QUINOA ARE CREATED EQUAL!
Since the ancient super nutritious, faux grain quinoa conquered the world it's become a huge industry in its home countries of Peru and Bolivia, bringing wealth and development to the natives. But it's not a totally sunny story. The massive rise in demand has lead to rocketing prices, meaning many locals are unable to afford quinoa themselves. The intense production, with its reliance on toxic pesticides and chemicals, has also depleted the farmland. Choosing organic Fairtrade quinoa ensures that the the local producers are working to reduce the impact on the environment and paying fair wages.

SERVES 4
1 cup quinoa

SALSA
bunch of heirloom cherry tomatoes or tomatillos, finely diced
1 white or red onion, finely diced
1 red bell pepper, finely diced
juice of 1 lime

BAJA SAUCE
$^2/_3$ cup sour cream
juice of 1 lime
pinch of salt

SPICY BEANS
olive oil
2 shallots, diced
$14^1/_2$ oz. can beans, rinsed and drained
$2^1/_2$ cups Le Puy lentils, cooked
1 teaspoon ground or fresh oregano
2 garlic cloves, finely chopped to a paste
$^1/_2$ teaspoon cumin
1–2 jalapeño peppers, seeded and finely chopped
1 teaspoon paprika
$^3/_4$ teaspoon salt

SERVE WITH
2 avocados, pitted, peeled, and sliced
lime wedges
corn tortilla chips (optional)
hot sauce like Cholula or Sriracha
hemp seeds
bunch of spinach

Harvest Root Bowl

BARLEY WITH SWISS CHARD, ROASTED ROOTS, AND TARRAGON DRESSING

Beneath the rough exterior of root vegetables is rich flavor—and roasting brings out the best in all of them. This bowl gathers the delights of early autumn with aromatic herbs, deep-roasted roots, and a scrumptious grain—barley. This root bowl is a great base for all kinds of additions. Serve with crunchy toasted nuts, or a soft cheese like feta or goat cheese.

Preheat the oven to 375°F and line a baking sheet with parchment. Cook the barley according to the package instructions. Drain and set aside.

Chop the root vegetables into even-sized chunks to ensure they roast uniformly. Put all the veggies and shallots on the lined baking sheet and drizzle with olive oil. Sprinkle with the sage and salt. Roast for 35 to 40 minutes.

Bring a saucepan of water to a boil, then turn down the heat to a simmer. Cook the stems of the chard for 90 seconds, remove, and rinse under ice cold water. Blanch the leaves of the Swiss chard for 30 seconds, remove, and rinse under ice cold water.

Blend the ingredients for the tarragon dressing and set aside until ready to serve. Divide the barley, roasted roots, and Swiss chard between four serving bowls. Serve with the tarragon dressing and cheese or nuts.

VE *Use vegan cheese if adding.*
GF *Substitute buckwheat for barley.*

SERVES 4
1 cup hulled or pearl barley
1 lb. mixed root vegetables (fennel, beets, carrots, sweet potato), washed, trimmed, and peeled
4 shallots, halved
olive oil, for roasting
handful of fresh sage leaves, finely chopped
bunch of Swiss chard, stems separated from leaves, chopped

TARRAGON DRESSING
1/2 cup extra-virgin olive oil
1 teaspoon Dijon mustard
1 tablespoon tarragon leaves
1 teaspoon honey
juice of 1/2 lemon
1 garlic clove, finely chopped to a paste

SUGGESTED TOPPINGS
8 oz. feta or goat cheese
toasted hazelnuts or almonds

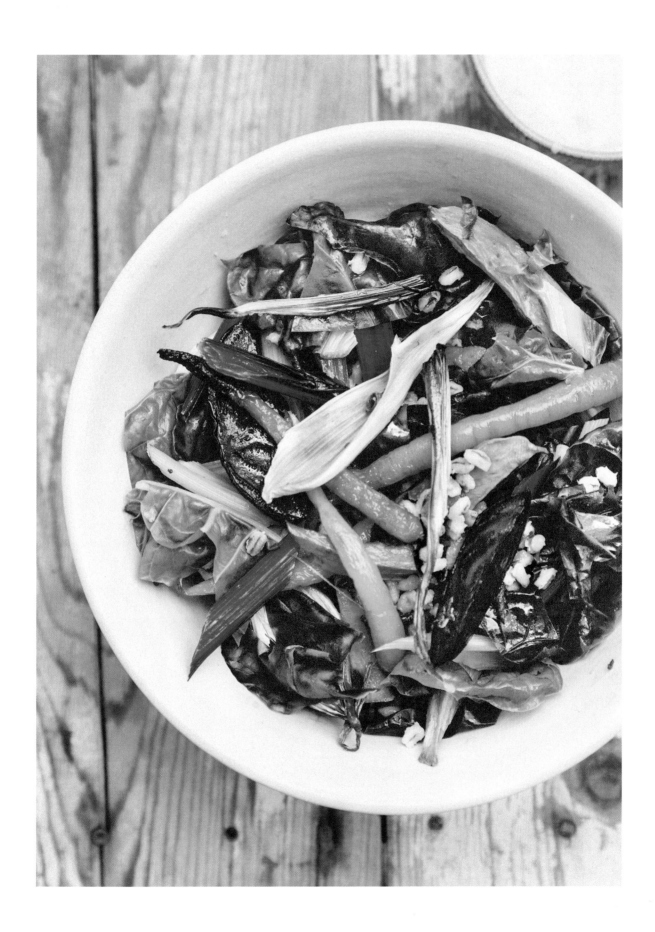

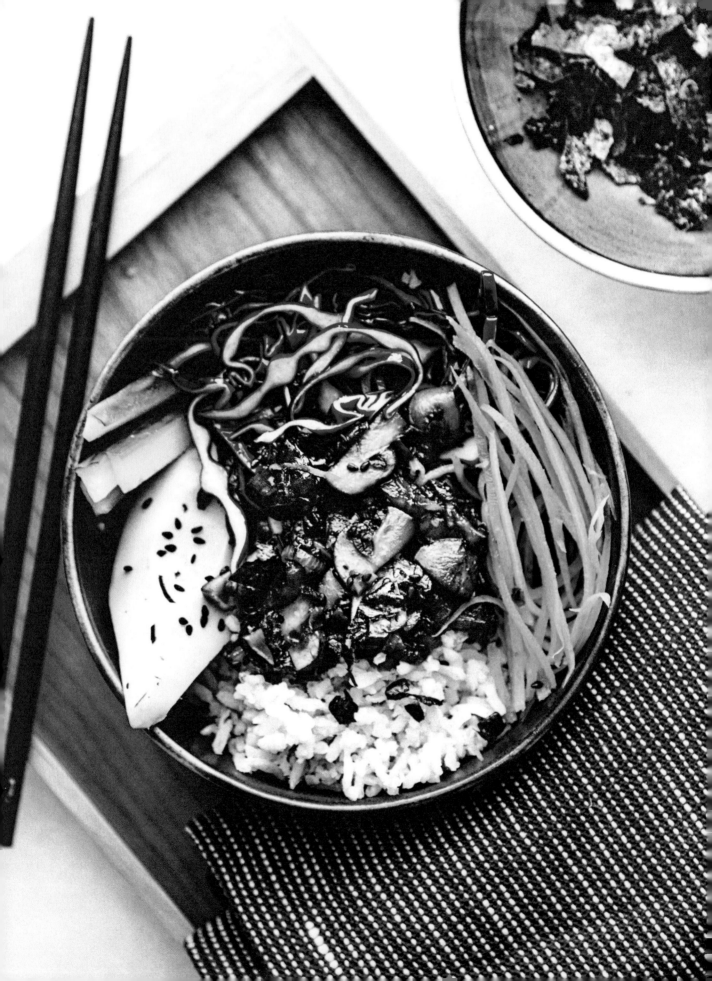

Donburi

JAPANESE RICE BOWL WITH EGGPLANT, SHIITAKE MUSHROOMS, AND QUICK-PICKLED CABBAGE

Donburi is a popular everyday comfort bowl in Japan and one of the most common lunch dishes. It's usually based on rice and topped with meat or vegetables. The sauce is reminiscent of teriyaki sauce and it makes the perfect sweet and savory union with the sautéed eggplant and mushrooms. Plain freshly cooked rice doesn't get better than this, soaking up a sauce full of flavor. Adding pickled cabbage and fresh carrot and cucumber makes a perfect balance of sour, sweet, and savory in this delicious, easy bowl.

Cook the rice according to the package instructions. Place the cabbage in a bowl. Mix the rice vinegar, toasted sesame oil, and agave syrup in a small bowl, Pour over the cabbage and toss to coat. Set aside to pickle.

Mix the ingredients for the donburi sauce in a small bowl.

Heat a skillet over medium-high heat and add a drizzle of olive oil. Cook the eggplant, mushrooms, and shallots for 5 minutes, stirring. Add the donburi sauce and cook 5 minutes more, still stirring.

Divide the rice and the cooked vegetables between four serving bowls. Add the pickled cabbage, cucumber, carrots, and avocado. Mix the nori and sesame sprinkle ingredients in a small bowl and scatter over the donburi before serving.

VE ✓

GF *Use gluten-free tamari instead of soy sauce.*

SERVES 4

1 cup brown rice
1 cup shredded red or white cabbage
drizzle of rice vinegar
drizzle of toasted sesame oil
1 teaspoon agave syrup
olive oil, for sauteing
1 eggplant, chopped small
2/3 lb. shiitake or brown mushrooms, chopped
4 shallots, chopped
1/2 cucumber, cut into matchsticks
2 carrots, julienned
1 avocado, pitted, peeled, and sliced

DONBURI SAUCE

1/3 cup soy sauce
1/4 cup mirin
1 tablespoon maple syrup
1/2 teaspoon freshly grated ginger
1 garlic clove, finely chopped to a paste
salt and pepper

NORI AND SESAME SPRINKLE

handful of toasted nori flakes
1 tablespoon shichimi togarashi
handful of black sesame seeds

Gado Gado

EGG, TEMPEH, AND BLACK COCONUT RICE WITH PEANUT SAUCE AND PAPAYA

Amsterdam is a great place to enjoy Indonesian cuisine. Since Colonial times, Dutch food culture has been enriched by the vibrant cooking of Indonesian immigrants. One of my Indonesian favorites is gado gado, a rice bowl drizzled with a delicious peanut sauce.

In this recipe I'm using highly nutritious black rice, also called "forbidden rice"–the name by which it was known in ancient China when only the Emperor was allowed to eat it. Luckily, today we can all enjoy black rice in this delectable bowl!

Blend the ingredients for the gado gado sauce together. Add water to thin to your desired consistency. Mix the marinade ingredients together in a bowl. Add the tempeh pieces, refrigerate, and let marinate, covered, for at least 45 minutes.

Place the black rice in a large saucepan with the kaffir lime leaves and 2 cups water. Bring to a boil, then turn down the heat. Let it simmer for 20 to 30 minutes if you pre-soaked it, or 50 minutes if you didn't. To avoid over-cooking your rice, begin checking it early. Once cooked, remove the lime leaves and drain the rice, then transfer to a bowl.

Meanwhile, bring another saucepan of water to a boil. Place the eggs in the saucepan with the green beans and a good pinch of salt. Simmer for 6 minutes, then remove from the heat and transfer the eggs and green beans into ice-cold water to chill. Drain and set aside.

Toast the shredded coconut in a dry skillet, stirring until golden brown. Remove from the heat and mix half the toasted coconut with the black rice and season with salt.

Divide the rice between four serving bowls along with the bean sprouts, green beans, and papaya. Remove the tempeh pieces from the marinade and fry over medium-high heat for 2 to 3 minutes on each side. Add the tempeh to the serving bowls and drizzle generously with gado gado sauce. Top with the eggs (peeled and halved), fresh cilantro, and the remaining toasted coconut.

VE *Omit the eggs for a vegan meal.*
GF *Use gluten-free tamari instead of soy sauce.*

SERVES 4

8 oz. tempeh, cut into pieces
1 cup black rice, pre-soaked for 3 hours
handful of kaffir lime leaves
4 eggs
bunch of green beans
3$\frac{1}{4}$ cup shredded coconut
2 handfuls of bean sprouts
$\frac{1}{2}$ papaya, peeled and seeded, cut into small wedges
handful of cilantro leaves
salt

GADO GADO SAUCE

$\frac{1}{3}$ cup natural peanut butter
2 tablespoons tamarind paste
1 tablespoon coconut sugar
juice of 1 lime
$\frac{1}{4}$ cup soy sauce

MARINADE

generous drizzle of sesame oil
2 garlic cloves, finely chopped to a paste
1 tablespoon freshly grated ginger
1 tablespoon maple syrup
$\frac{1}{4}$ cup soy sauce
1$\frac{1}{2}$ tablespoons Sriracha

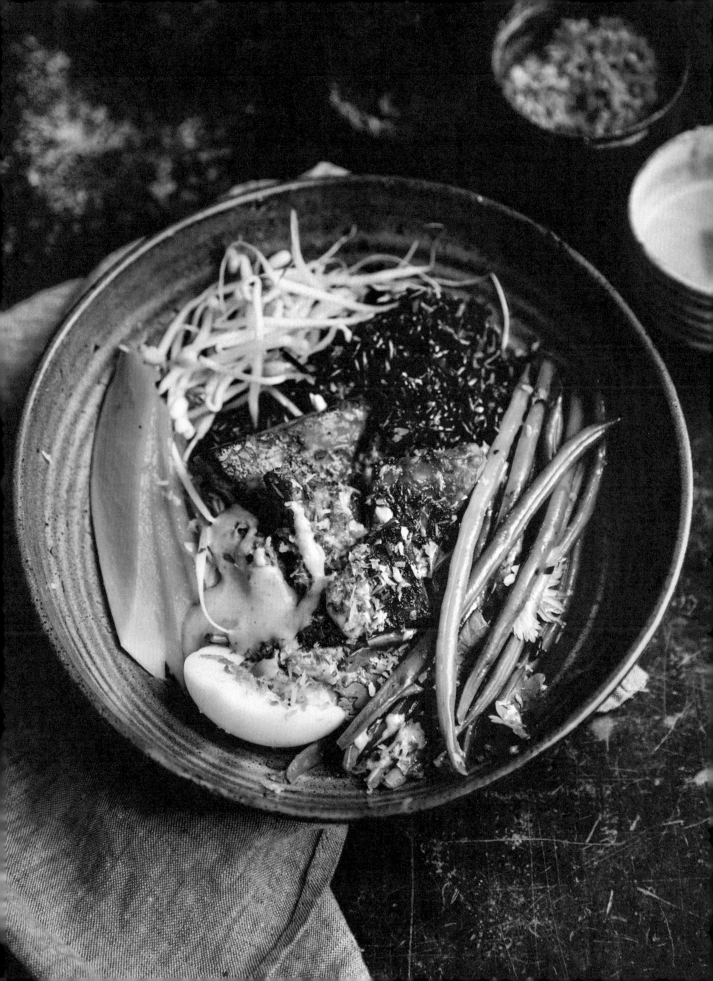

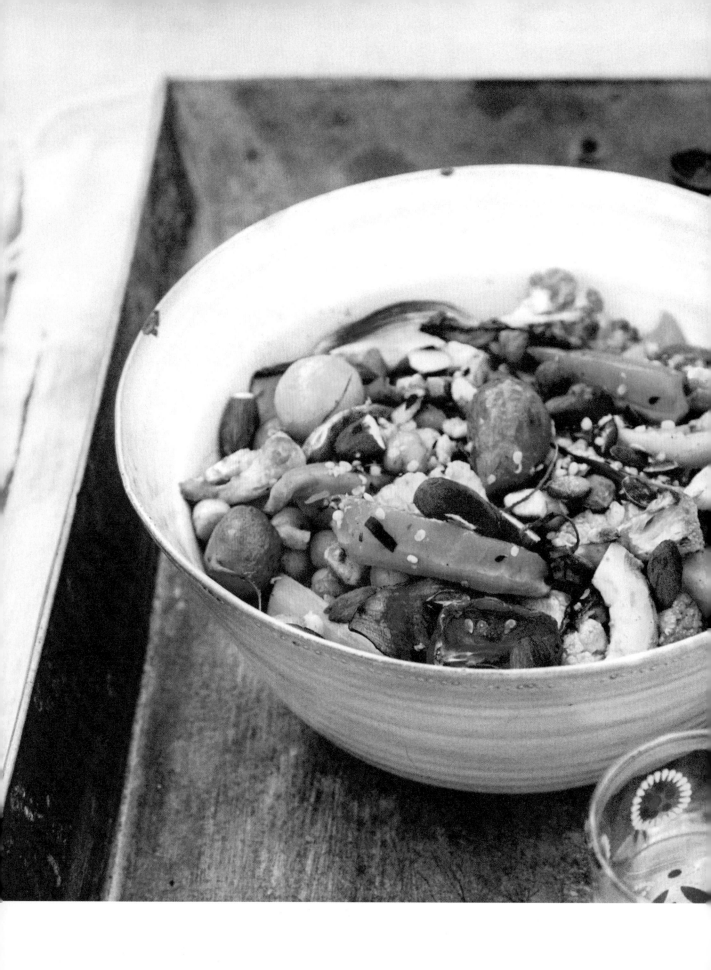

Masala and Millet Bowl

GARAM MASALA AND CARDAMOM ROASTED VEGETABLES WITH FLUFFY MILLET

Cinnamon and cardamom add a comforting quality to this roasted vegetable and millet bowl, while garam masala gives a distinct Indian flavor to the vegetables. This bowl is a crowd pleaser. Serve with the herbed yogurt sauce and top with crunchy toasted nuts.

Preheat the oven to 400°F and line a baking sheet with parchment. Cook the millet according to the package instructions. Drain and set aside to dry before serving.

Place the vegetables and chickpeas on the prepared baking sheet. Mix the ground spices with the olive oil, then drizzle over the vegetables. Rub the spiced oil into the veggies, season with salt, and roast for 40 to 45 minutes. Turn the vegetables over halfway through cooking and keep a close eye in the last 15 minutes.

Mix the ingredients for the herbed yogurt into a smooth sauce and refrigerate until ready to serve.

Fluff the millet with a fork in a large bowl and mix with the roasted vegetables and chickpeas. Add the avocado and top with toasted nuts and seeds. Serve with the herbed yogurt sauce.

Tip! You can vary the grain and choice of vegetables with similar ingredients.

VE *Use vegan yogurt instead of Greek yogurt.*
GF ✓

SERVES 4

1 cup millet
1–2 lbs. mixed vegetables to roast
  (carrots, radishes, cauliflower,
  red onion, bell peppers, and
  tomatoes, cut in small pieces)
8 oz. can chickpeas
1/4 cup olive oil
1 teaspoon garam masala
3/4 teaspoon ground cardamom
1/2 teaspoon cinnamon
1/4 teaspoon cayenne pepper
1/2 teaspoon paprika
salt
2 avocados, pitted, peeled,
  and sliced
1 cup mixed nuts and seeds of your
  choice, such as toasted almonds,
  pumpkin seeds, or hemp seeds

HERBED YOGURT SAUCE
  (makes about 3/4 cup)
1 cup Greek yogurt
juice of 1/2 lemon
handful of chopped mint
1/2 teaspoon ground coriander
1 garlic clove, finely chopped
  to a paste
3 tablespoons olive oil
1 teaspoon agave syrup

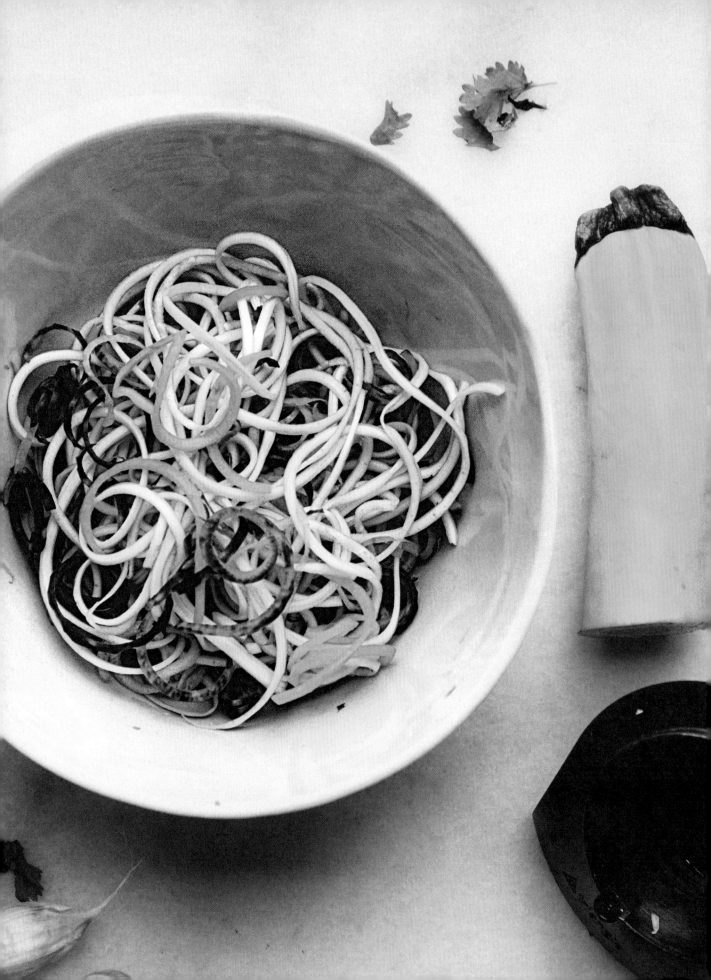

ZOODLES, NOODLES, AND PASTA

Tangles, threads, ribbons, and little shells—how we love them
for soaking up sauces and for layering with delicious flavors. There's
a wealth of noodles and pastas to choose from, made from
a variety of flours and vegetables. It's also fun to make your own.
Raw vegetable noodles add juiciness to both Italian- and Asian-style dishes.
Zoodles have become quite a phenomenon on
gluten-free and healthy food blogs. Rice, spelt, and buckwheat
make delicious alternatives to refined wheat pasta.
My personal favorite is the soba noodle, made from buckwheat
flour, which is delectable in both warm and cold dishes.

Velvet Tagliatelle

HANDMADE SPELT AND BEET PASTA

Making your own pasta is incredibly easy. It's all about kneading your flour to a silky smooth dough. These strands of tagliatelle are velvet-hued too, from the natural color of beets. What I love most about homemade pasta is the imperfection—that handmade touch and rustic look—and the fresh flavor is heavenly!

This pasta dough can be used for different shapes of pasta and served with a variety of sauces. It's made with spelt flour, an ancient protein-rich grain that contains less gluten than wheat and has a delicious, nutty flavor. The beauty of fresh pasta is that it doesn't need much to shine; serve it with salt, pepper, olive oil, and garlic, with a simple pesto, or just sprinkled with Parmesan.

Shape the flour into a tall heap on a work surface, then create a deep well in the middle. Crack the eggs into the well and add the beet juice. Little by little, bring the flour into the middle and mix with the liquid ingredients using a fork. Add more flour if needed. Knead the dough for 5 to 10 minutes, then form into a ball and cover with plastic wrap. Let rest for 30 minutes.

After the dough has rested, dust the work surface with flour and knead for a few more minutes. Roll out until the dough is paper thin, working in batches if necessary. If the dough is too sticky, dust more flour on the surface and roll out again.

Using a knife or a pasta cutter, cut long thin strands of tagliatelle. Place the tagliatelle on a sheet of parchment to dry for 30 minutes. The pasta can then be stored sealed in the fridge for a couple of days.

When you are ready to cook the pasta, bring a large saucepan of water to a boil. Reduce the heat to a simmer, and add 1 tablespoon of olive oil and 1 teaspoon of salt, then the tagliatelle. Cook for 1 to 3 minutes, then drain. Serve with your choice of sauce or simply with basil leaves, salt, pepper, ricotta flavored with a crushed garlic clove, and extra-virgin olive oil.

Tip! Make regular tagliatelle by omitting the beet juice and using ⅓ cup less spelt flour.

VE *The texture and bite will be less silky for the vegan version: replace each egg with 4 tablespoons water.*

GF *This recipe is not gluten-free.*

SERVES 4

PASTA
1 lb. spelt flour, plus extra
   for dusting
4 eggs
½ cup raw beet juice
1 tablespoon olive oil
1 teaspoon salt

TO SERVE
handful of basil leaves
extra-virgin olive oil
½ cup ricotta
1 garlic clove, finely chopped
   to a paste
salt and pepper

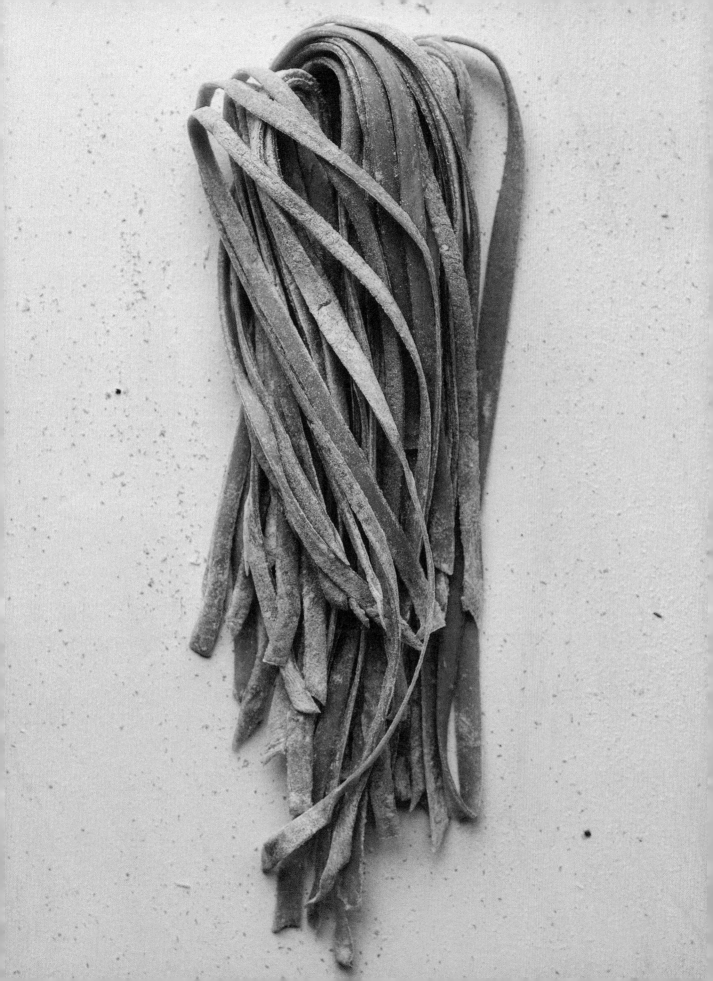

Grilled Eggplant and Pappardelle

HOMEMADE WHOLE-GRAIN SPELT PASTA WITH GRILLED EGGPLANT AND LEMON

Made with layers of juicy roasted vegetables, this pasta captures the flavor of rustic southern Italian cooking. Tomatoes and eggplants are sun-worshipping plants, adding a warm sweetness to the garlic and lemon tang of this dish. A little cardamom gives a hint of Morocco. A real sunshine bowl!

Preheat the oven to 425°F. For the pappardelle, follow the recipe for tagliatelle on page 108 but use 1 ounce less flour and omit the beet juice. Use a knife to cut long, wide strands of pasta.

Arrange the eggplants, tomatoes, garlic, red onions, and scallions on a baking sheet lined with parchment. Drizzle with olive oil, sprinkle with salt and thyme, and roast for 15 minutes.

Meanwhile, cook the pasta according to the package instructions or according to page 108 if you've made your own. Drain, reserving a little of the pasta water in the bottom of the pot.

Remove the vegetables from the oven and transfer them to a large skillet. Drizzle with vinegar and lemon juice and sprinkle with ground cardamom. Cook slowly over medium-low heat for 5 minutes. Add the pasta with the reserved pasta water and toss with the roasted veggies for 2 to 3 minutes. Season with salt and pepper to taste. Drizzle with extra-virgin olive oil and serve with grated pecorino and basil leaves.

VE *Use rawmesan instead of pecorino*
    or omit cheese.
GF *Choose a gluten-free pasta.*

SERVES 4

8 oz. papardelle (see tagliatelle, page 108)
2 eggplants, cut into bite-size pieces
1/2 lb. heirloom tomatoes, halved or quartered, depending on size
2 garlic cloves, thinly sliced
2 red onions, cut in wedges
4 scallions, halved lengthwise
2 tablespoons fresh thyme
drizzle of red wine vinegar
juice of 1/2 lemon
sprinkle of ground cardamom
olive oil
salt and pepper

TO SERVE

extra-virgin olive oil
pecorino or rawmesan (page 53)
basil leaves

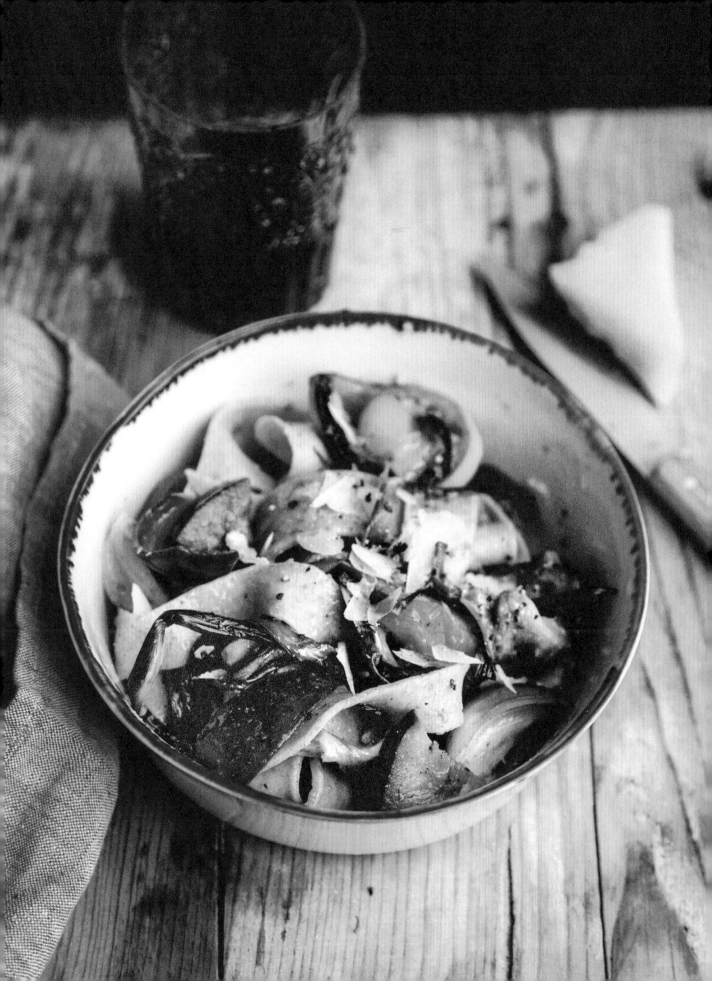

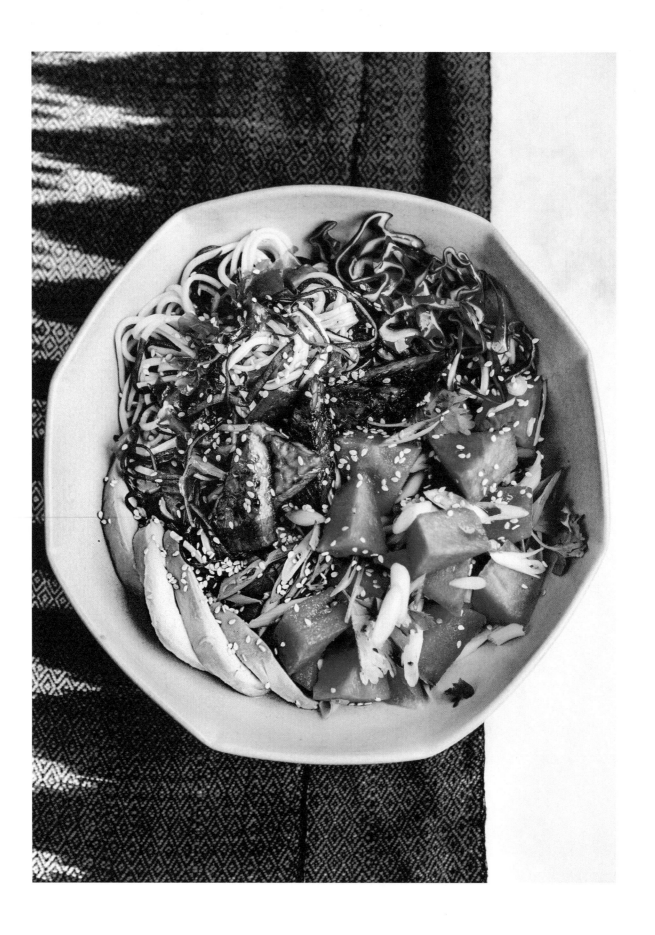

Watermelon Poke Bowl

SOBA NOODLES, WATERMELON, SEAWEED, TEMPEH WITH A ZESTY GINGER DRESSING

Aloha! Tuna poke bowls are increasingly popular outside the Hawaiian kitchen. My favorite vegetarian version of this dish is made with watermelon and seaweed for the acquatic flavor. Even with no fish, these ingredients give a taste of the sea. This poke noodle bowl makes an easy and satisfying meal, as well as providing a bundle of goodness, with fermented tempeh, avocado, seaweed, and buckwheat soba noodles. Soba noodles are delicious cold and here they are coated with a wonderful ginger and soy dressing. Like tofu, tempeh is made from soybeans but it has a bit more bite. It's perfect marinated and fried. This bowl is easily prepared using prepped ingredients, making it ideal for quick lunches and weekday meals.

Mix the marinade ingredients in a bowl, add the tempeh and toss gently to coat, then cover with plastic wrap and refrigerate for at least 30 minutes.

Mix the dressing ingredients and set aside until ready to serve.

Meanwhile, cook the soba noodles according to the package instructions. Drain, rinse under cold water, and set aside.

Place the seaweed in a bowl and cover with water. Soak for 10 minutes, then drain and toss with the cold soba noodles.

Toss the watermelon pieces with cilantro and scallion. Heat a skillet over medium-high heat, add a tablespoon of coconut oil, and fry the tempeh triangles until they're nicely browned.

Divide the soba noodles between four serving bowls and top with the cabbage, avocado, watermelon, and tempeh. Serve with the dressing and a sprinkle of sesame seeds.

VE ✓

GF *Use gluten-free tamari instead of soy sauce.*

SERVES 4

8 oz. tempeh, cut into 2–3 slices about 1/2-inch thick, then into triangles
10 oz. soba noodles
2 handfuls of dulse (or your choice of seaweed)
2 handfuls Irish sea spaghetti (or your choice of seaweed)
1 1/2 lbs. watermelon, peeled, seeded, and cut into bite-size pieces
2 handfuls of cilantro, roughly chopped
3 scallions, finely sliced
1 1/2 cups finely shredded red cabbage
2 avocados, pitted, peeled, and sliced into wedges
sesame seeds
coconut oil
salt and pepper

MARINADE

1 teaspoon freshly grated ginger
3 tablespoons soy sauce
1 garlic clove, finely chopped to a paste
1 teaspoon hot sauce, such as Sriracha
1 teaspoon agave syrup

GINGER DRESSING

zest and juice of 1 lime
1 teaspoon freshly grated ginger
1 tablespoon rice vinegar
1/4 cup soy sauce
2 tablespoons extra-virgin olive oil
1 teaspoon hot sauce, such as Sriracha

1 tablespoon toasted sesame seeds

Bread Crumb Chitarra

SPAGHETTI WITH MUDDICA, BABY SPINACH, AND GARLIC

There are many things you learn when you first move away from home. I became a master of minimalist pastas that require only a few ingredients, which was very handy since stocking up the kitchen wasn't a priority in my student days. Today I still love the easy but genius ways of cooking a simple pasta dish. Herbs, olive oil, lemon, salt, pepper, and Parmesan go a long way, but my most unexpected favorite is bread crumbs. A bread crumb topping on pasta, or *muddica* as it's called in Italian, is a beloved everyday sprinkle in Sicily and it's growing in popularity elsewhere as a vegan alternative to Parmesan. But not just for vegans. Foodies unite behind the brilliance of simple bread crumbs—poor man's Parmesan—with a little flavoring from garlic and lemon. It is delicious on salads and soups as well.

This pasta bowl is enriched with nourishing baby spinach, which adds a delicious taste. *Chitarra* means guitar and for this dish you can use any long-stranded pasta or noodles.

Cook the pasta according to the package instructions. Drain, reserving a little of the cooking water, then season with salt, and drizzle with extra-virgin olive oil.

Meanwhile, to make the muddica, heat a skillet over medium-high heat and add the olive oil. Stir in the garlic and cook for a few seconds. Add the bread crumbs and fry until golden brown, 3 to 4 minutes. Remove from the heat, add the salt and lemon zest, and transfer to a bowl.

Reheat the pan and add a drizzle of olive oil. Cook the baby spinach for 1 minute until wilted, then add the pasta, and mix with the spinach. Add salt and pepper to taste. Serve in bowls topped with the muddica and a little lemon zest.

VE *This recipe is vegan.*
GF *Use gluten-free pasta and bread crumbs.*

SERVES 4

12 oz. chitarra (or long-stranded pasta of your choice, such as gluten-free, or whole-grain spelt)
extra-virgin olive oil
2 cups baby spinach
salt and pepper

MUDDICA
1/4 cup olive oil
2 garlic cloves, finely chopped to a paste
2 cups bread crumbs (use fresh or dry bread)
1 teaspoon salt
1 teaspoon lemon zest and extra for topping

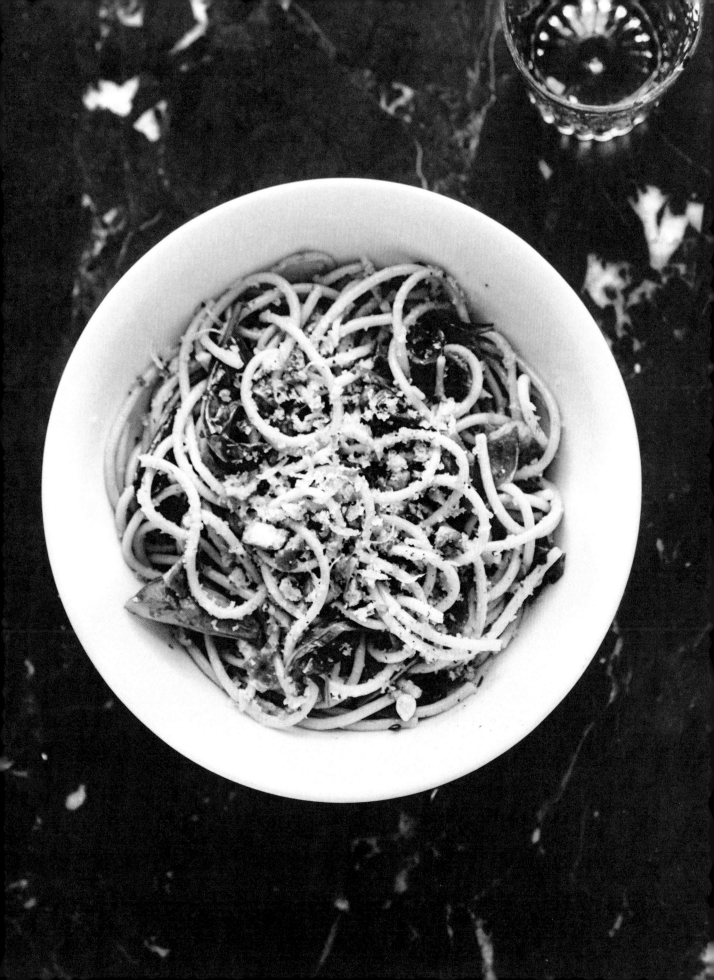

Laksa Noodles

RICE NOODLES WITH VEGETABLES AND LEMONGRASS COCONUT SAUCE

In this dish, a Malaysian laksa of lemongrass and coconut milk provides a fragrant tangy base for spicy tofu and veggies. Lemongrass has a mild citrus flavor that adds freshness to food, here offering a perfect balance to the mushrooms, eggs, and onions. The bouncy rice noodles give a neutral smooth finish. You can vary the steamed vegetables and swap the tofu for other proteins such as beans. As it's both refreshing and comforting, it's an ideal noodle bowl all year around.

Preheat the oven to its lowest setting. To make the pickle, put the cucumber and red onion in a small bowl, and drizzle with the rice vinegar. Set aside until ready to serve.

Put all the ingredients for the laksa paste into a food processor and blend until smooth.

Heat a skillet over medium-high heat and add a tablespoon of coconut oil. Cook the tofu for 2 to 3 minutes, stirring carefully, until crisp. Season with salt and red pepper flakes, and fry for another minute. Transfer the tofu to a baking sheet and keep warm in the oven.

Wipe out the skillet, reheat over medium-high heat, and melt another tablespoon of coconut oil. Sauté the mushrooms for 3 to 4 minutes. Season with salt and pepper to taste. Transfer the mushrooms to a small bowl and keep warm in the oven.

Steam the broccoli and green beans for 3 to 4 minutes, after 2 minutes of steaming add the bean sprouts. Remove from the heat and set aside, covered.

Wipe out the skillet, reheat over medium-high heat and melt a third tablespoon of coconut oil. Cook the laksa paste for a minute, using a wooden spoon to break it up gently in the pan. Add the vegetable broth, lime juice, and coconut milk and stir to dissolve the paste into the liquid. Let it simmer for 4 to 5 minutes. Season with salt and pepper and keep warm.

Cook the rice noodles according to the package instructions and drain. Divide the noodles, mushrooms, steamed veggies, tofu, and egg halves between serving bowls and top with pickles. Pour laksa sauce over the bowls and sprinkle with sesame seeds. Serve immediately. Serve with Sriracha, sesame oil, lime wedges, fresh cilantro, and any remaining laksa sauce.

VE *Omit the eggs.*

GF *Use gluten-free tamari instead of soy sauce.*

SERVES 4

7 oz. firm tofu, pressed (see page 16) and cut into small cubes
coconut oil
1 teaspoon salt
1 teaspoon red pepper flakes
3/4 lb. mushrooms, cleaned and sliced
small head broccoli, florets only
1/2 lb. green beans
1/2 lb. fresh bean sprouts
3 cups vegetable broth (see page 56)
juice of 1 lime
14 oz. can coconut milk
8 oz. rice noodles
4 boiled eggs (cooked for 7 minutes), peeled and halved
sesame seeds
salt and pepper

PICKLE

1/2 cucumber, shaved into ribbons
1 red onion, finely sliced
rice vinegar for sushi

LAKSA SPICE PASTE (REMPAH)

2 tablespoons finely chopped fresh lemongrass
1 tablespoon freshly grated ginger
3 garlic cloves, crushed
2 tablespoons sambal oelek
4 shallots, finely chopped
1 tablespoon freshly grated turmeric
1 tablespoon toasted sesame oil
3 tablespoons soy sauce
2 tablespoons coconut sugar
2 tablespoons vegetable oil

TO SERVE

Sriracha, sesame oil, lime wedges, fresh cilantro

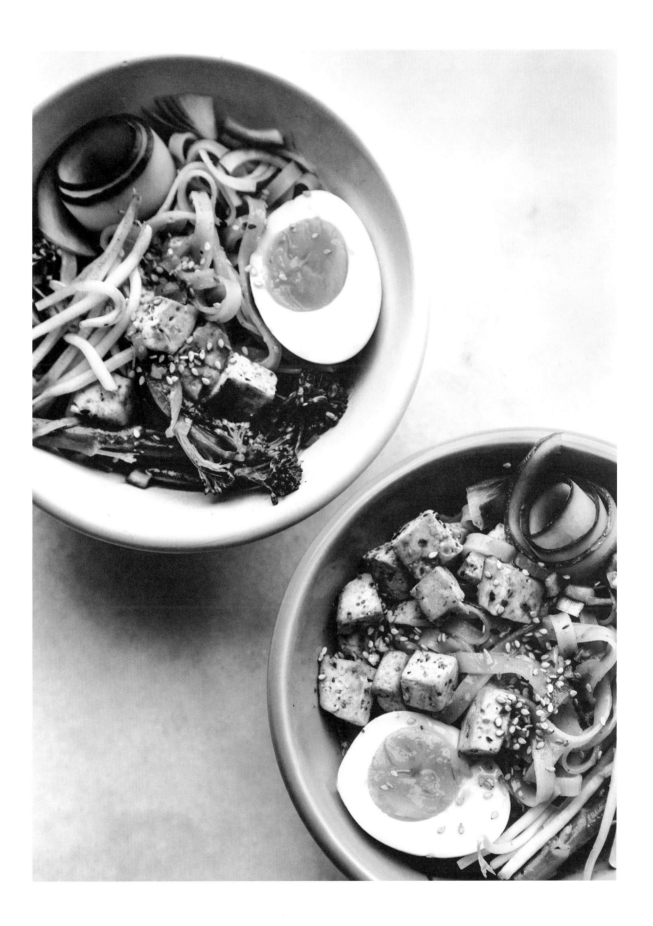

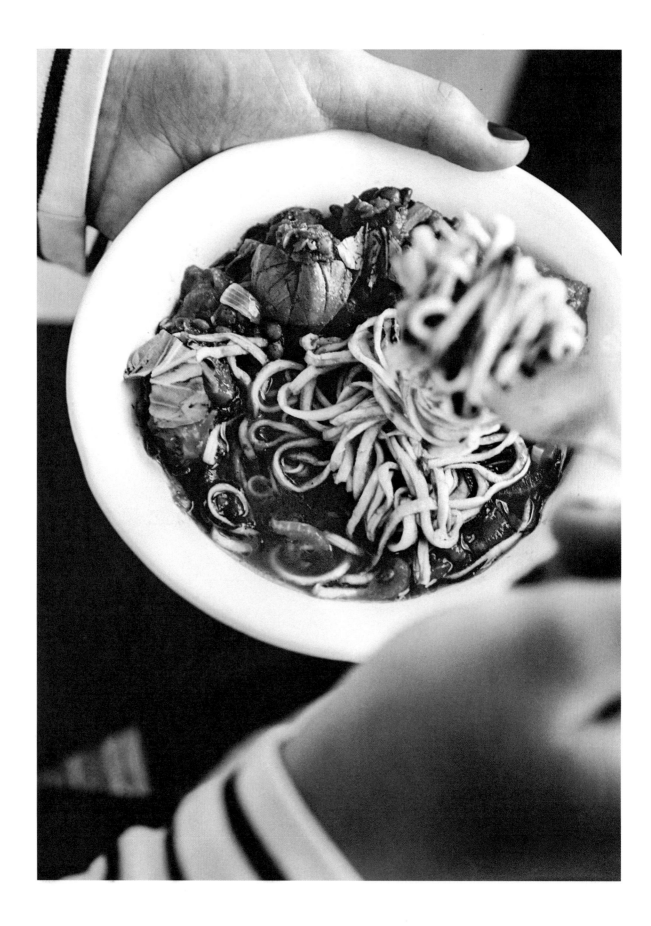

Lentil Ragu and Zoodles

SUPER DELICIOUS, PLANT-BASED VERSION OF SPAGHETTI BOLOGNESE!

Lentil ragu is as popular with vegetarian families as Bolognese is with carnivores. No one can resist it. Served with a bowl of zoodles—the zucchini version of raw spiralized noodle strands—it makes the perfect healthy comfort meal. Zoodles are not just a gluten-free, skinny pasta alternative, they're so delicious you'll be wanting to enjoy them with all sorts of sauces.

Bring 4 cups water to a boil in a large saucepan. Add the lentils and simmer for 30 to 35 minutes until soft. Drain, rinse in cold water, and set aside.

Heat a skillet over medium-high heat and add a drizzle of olive oil. Cook the chopped vegetables and mushrooms until fragrant and the shallots are translucent. Add the drained lentils and garlic-salt paste and stir. Drizzle in the vinegar and add the chopped tomatoes and honey to the pan. Sprinkle with marjoram and simmer for a few minutes, adding water if necessary. Taste and adjust with salt and pepper. Divide ragu with zoodles in serving bowls and serve with sprinkles of Parmesan or rawmesan and fresh herbs.

VE *Use rawmesan (see page 53) and agave syrup instead of honey.*

GF ✓

SERVES 4

olive oil
1 cup Le Puy lentils
1 carrot, finely chopped
1 celery stalk, finely chopped
4 shallots, finely chopped
$\frac{1}{4}$ lb. mushrooms, finely chopped
2 garlic cloves, finely chopped
   to a paste with 1 teaspoon salt
2 tablespoons red wine vinegar
14$\frac{1}{2}$ oz. can diced tomatoes
1 teaspoon honey or agave syrup
1 tablespoon marjoram leaves
2 zucchini, spiralized
salt and pepper

TO SERVE

Parmesan or rawmesan
   (see page 53)
fresh herbs

SPIRALIZED VEGGIES: *It's becoming increasingly popular to spiralize, a delicious way to eat more vegetables. You can spiralize almost any firm vegetable (root veggies and zucchini are especially suited). Carrots make tasty tagliatelle and daikon makes firm and bouncy noodles. There's a variety of tools to use, I own both a cheap small cone with a blade and a machine that was a bit more pricey but the cone works better! You can also use a cheese slicer or peeler and a knife for tagliatelle.*

Polpette with Garden Pesto

VEGGIE NEATBALLS WITH BASIL, DILL, AND SPINACH SAUCE

This "amazeballs" pasta dish is your regular meatball and pasta turned into a lusher green version. The pesto sauce is full of herbal flavor and so easy to make that I use it both cold and warm with all sorts of foods in addition to pasta—grilled vegetables, salads, potatoes. In the summer I go round all the herbs in the garden and grab a handful to blend with olive oil, salt, and lemon juice. In this recipe, I've added vegan crème fraîche (you can use dairy crème fraîche, too) for a creamier sauce.

Cook the pasta according to the package instructions, drain, but leave a little cooking water in the bottom of the saucepan. Blend the ingredients for the garden pesto sauce in a food processor and set aside. Follow the recipe for the neatballs on page 164. When you have finished frying the neatballs, transfer them to a low-temperature oven while heating the garden pesto sauce. Divide the pasta, sauce, and neatballs in serving bowls.

VE *Use vegan crème fraîche, and toppings. Choose egg-free pasta.*

GF *Choose gluten-free pasta and bread crumbs or panko for the neatballs.*

SERVES 4

GARDEN PESTO SAUCE
handful of fresh dill
small handful of mint leaves
2 handfuls of basil leaves
1–2 garlic cloves
¼ cup chopped leek
juice of ½ lemon
2 handfuls of baby spinach
¾ cup vegan or dairy crème fraîche
¼ cup extra-virgin olive oil
salt and pepper

TO SERVE
12 oz. pasta
30 neatballs (see page 164)

PRESERVING HERBS: *When herbs are growing in abundance, faster than you can enjoy them, extend the time you can use them in your cooking by turning to pesto making. Tender herbs such as basil, parsley, mint, and cilantro are better for pestos than the sturdier herbs, but mix and match according to taste. Chop as fine as you can—the flavors are hidden in the cellulose of the plants and the finer they are minced, the more flavor is released. Olive oil and a little salt further enhance the flavor of the herbs. That's the very simplest and purest type of pesto to make. From there on you can add ground nuts, lemon juice, grated Parmesan, or nutritional yeast for more interest.*

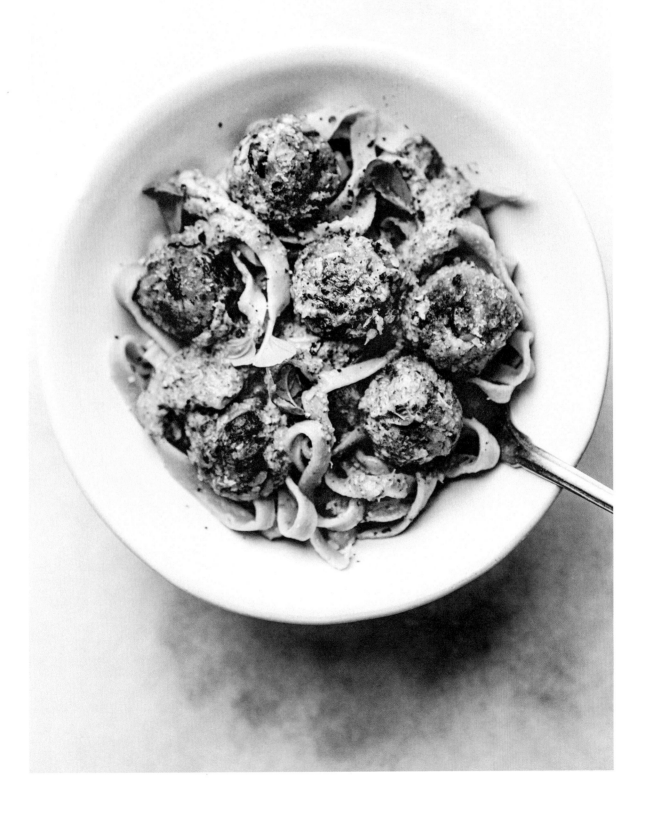

Slutty Pasta!

ROASTED TOMATO PUTTANESCA AND WHOLE-GRAIN SPELT SPAGHETTI

Pasta puttanesca is a famous Italian dish of tomatoes combined with a few strong, salty ingredients such as garlic, capers, and olives. Its origins involved making a dish of scraps found on hand in the kitchen, hence its unflattering name (puttanesca means prostitute-style). My "slutty pasta" deviates from the original recipe for the sauce by roasting the tomatoes beforehand, elevating its flavors to a more intense sweet juiciness.

Preheat the oven to 325°F. Put the tomatoes, red onions, and garlic on a baking sheet. Drizzle generously with olive oil and sprinkle with salt. Transfer the baking sheet to the oven and roast for 35 minutes.

Meanwhile, bring 2 liters of water to a boil in a large saucepan. Add ½ tablespoon salt and drizzle with olive oil. Cook the pasta for 1 to 2 minutes less than the recommended time on the package. Once cooked, measure out ⅔ cup of the pasta water for the tomato sauce. Drain the pasta, saving a little water in the saucepan to keep it from drying out. Set aside.

Remove the tomatoes from the oven. Reserve a few as a garnish and blend the rest of the tomatoes with the other sauce ingredients. Taste and adjust the seasoning with salt and pepper.

Heat a large skillet over medium-high heat and add the drained pasta and tomato sauce. Stir for 1 to 2 minutes with a wooden spoon to ensure the pasta is well coated. Taste and season with salt and pepper. Divide between bowls, add the reserved roasted tomatoes, and serve immediately with any of the suggested toppings.

VE *Use egg-free pasta and rawmesan.*
GF *Use gluten-free pasta.*

SERVES 2
6 oz. whole-grain spaghetti or
  pasta of choice

SAUCE
15 small tomatoes, halved
2 red onions
3 garlic cloves
olive oil
¼ cup black olives, pitted
⅔ cup reserved pasta cooking water
1 tablespoon red wine vinegar
1 teaspoon red pepper flakes
handful of basil leaves
salt and pepper

TOPPING SUGGESTIONS
toasted bread crumbs, Parmesan
  or rawmesan (see page 53), or
  crushed nuts and herbs

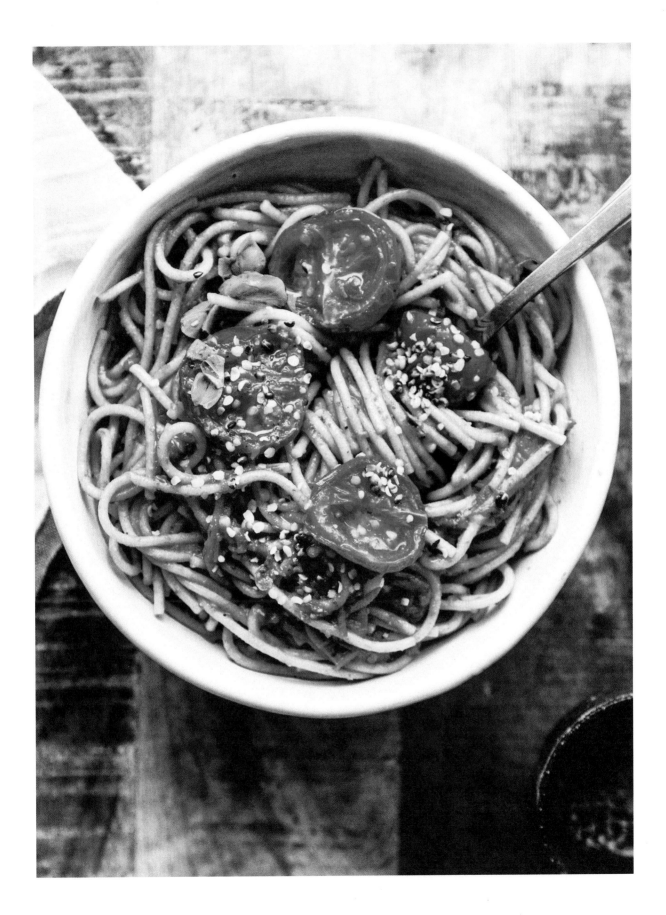

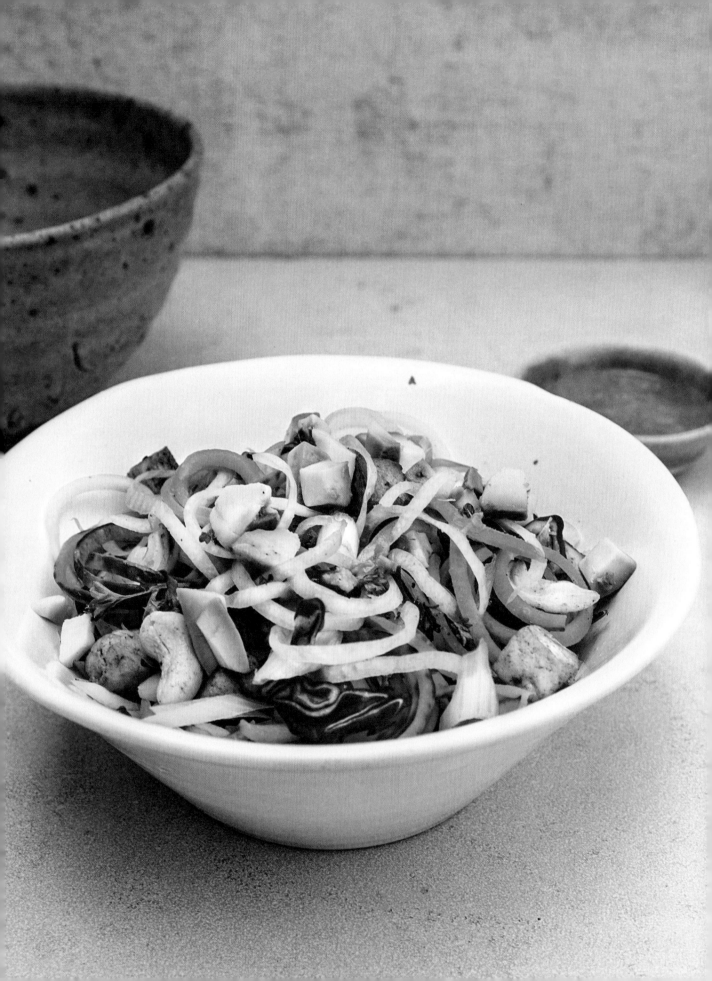

Rainbow Pad Thai

ALMOST-RAW RAINBOW CARROT NOODLES, TOASTED CASHEWS, AND SPICY TOFU

My family loves noodles in all shapes and colors. Serving a rainbow pad Thai pleases both small and grown-up eaters. It's a little juicier and fresher then regular rice or buckwheat noodles, so it complements the spicy tofu and peanut sauce beautifully. The avocado plays an important role here, adding a buttery creaminess that binds it all together. This noodle bowl is just as good as dinner as it is a side salad.

Mix the ingredients for the spicy peanut sauce and set aside.

Mix the coconut sugar with soy sauce, olive oil, and Sriracha for the tofu. Heat a skillet over medium-high heat and add 2 tablespoons coconut oil. Fry the tofu until golden, 2 to 3 minutes, then pour in the soy mix and cook for another 2 minutes while stirring. Remove from the heat.

Add another tablespoon of coconut oil and stir-fry the cashews over medium-high heat for 2 to 3 minutes, then remove from the heat.

Mix the carrot noodles with the avocado, red cabbage, cilantro, cashews, scallions, and tofu. Serve with the spicy peanut sauce.

VE ✓
GF *Use gluten-free tamari instead of soy sauce.*

SERVES 4
1 tablespoon coconut oil
3 handfuls of cashews
6 rainbow carrots, spiralized
2 avocados, pitted, peeled, and roughly chopped
1/4 small red cabbage, shredded
handful of chopped cilantro
6 scallions, finely chopped

SOY TOFU
1/4 cup coconut sugar
1/4 cup soy sauce
3 tablespoons olive oil
1/2 tablespoon Sriracha
2 tablespoons coconut oil
7 oz. firm tofu, pressed (see page 16)

SPICY PEANUT SAUCE
1/4 cup peanut butter
1 garlic clove, finely chopped to a paste
1 teaspoon freshly grated ginger
2 tablespoons soy sauce
2 tablespoons agave syrup
2 tablespoons tamarind paste
juice of 1 lime

Creamy Avocado, Walnut, and Spelt Rigatoni

WHOLE-GRAIN PASTA WITH NO-FUSS DAIRY-FREE PASTA SAUCE

This pasta dish uses avocado and garlic as a cold creamy sauce, with walnuts and leek for crunch. It's so quick and easy to make—a real time saver. You can use any herbs and nuts, and add tomatoes or cheese as extras.

Cook the pasta according to the package instructions, then drain and set aside. Place the avocado in a food processor and blend with the garlic, a drizzle of extra-virgin olive oil, and lemon juice. Taste and adjust with salt and pepper. Serve with rigatoni and top with walnuts, leek, and parsley.

SERVES 4

12 oz. whole-grain spelt rigatoni
  or your choice of pasta
3 avocados, pitted and peeled
2 garlic cloves
extra-virgin olive oil
juice of 1 lemon
salt and pepper
1½ cups walnuts
½ leek, white part only, trimmed
  and sliced in thin rounds
2 handfuls of parsley, chopped

VE *This pasta is vegan if you omit dairy cheese.*
GF *Choose a gluten-free pasta.*

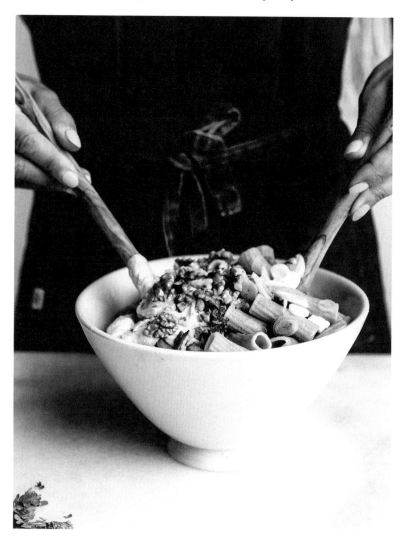

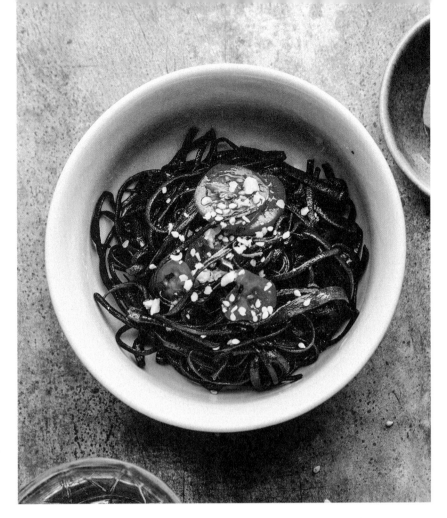

Frutti Di Mare

SEAWEED SPAGHETTI WITH TOMATOES AND GARLIC

The sea's own spaghetti makes a delicious starter. Irish seaweed spaghetti looks like pasta and tastes like the sea. It works beautifully with a little vinaigrette and tomato.

Rinse the seaweed. Bring a small pot of water to a boil, lower the heat, and add the seaweed. Let simmer for 5 minutes on low heat, then remove from heat and let it cool in the water for 30 minutes. Drain the seaweed and divide between four serving bowls. Slice the tomatoes and add to the bowls. Mix the dressing and drizzle over the seaweed. Serve sprinkled with sesame seeds.

VE ✓ GF ✓

JUST ENOUGH: *Although seaweed is super-nutritious, it should be eaten in moderation. Seaweed contains high levels of iodine that can be toxic in higher doses. Follow package instructions when you buy seaweed.*

SERVES 2
handful of Irish seaweed spaghetti
handful of cherry tomatoes
2 tablespoons sesame seeds

DRESSING
2 tablespoons extra-virgin olive oil
1 garlic clove, finely chopped
   to a paste
pinch of salt
2 tablespoons balsamic vinegar
½ tablespoon toasted sesame oil

Magic Mushroom Pasta

MUSHROOM PASTA WITH WHITE WINE, THYME, AND TARRAGON

Growing up, we picked mushrooms in the woods during autumn. When we got home, my parents were always happy to cook some right away and we would enjoy them on toast, fried with herbs. They tasted heavenly and I still love the aroma of fried mushrooms. In this scrumptious dish, mushrooms and herbs are balanced with the freshness of lemon and white wine. I often throw in a bunch of tarragon when I cook mushrooms—it's the perfect marriage. This pasta is a treat for dinner guests, but is so easy it makes a great weeknight supper, too.

Cook the pasta according to the package instructions. Drain, but leave some cooking water in the saucepan. Drizzle with a little olive oil.

Heat a skillet over medium-high heat. Add a drizzle of olive oil and arrange the mushrooms in the pan without overlapping. Cook until golden, about 3 minutes, turning the mushrooms and stirring frequently. Lightly season with salt and pepper. Add the garlic and herbs, with more olive oil if needed, and cook for 2 minutes. Add the pasta and wine and toss with the mushrooms, cooking for another minute. Season to taste and remove from heat. Serve with lemon zest, grated cheese or rawmesan, and a drizzle of olive oil.

VE *Use egg-free pasta; use rawmesan (page 53) or bread crumbs instead of Parmesan.*

GF *Choose a gluten-free pasta.*

SERVES 4

12 oz. tagliatelle (see page 108) or your choice of pasta

1 lb. mushrooms (a mix of chanterelle, brown, and shiitake), cleaned, large ones halved or quartered

2 garlic cloves, finely chopped to a paste

1 tablespoon chopped thyme leaves

1 teaspoon chopped tarragon leaves

$^1/_2$ cup dry white wine

extra-virgin olive oil

salt and pepper

TO SERVE

sprinkles of lemon zest

Parmesan or rawmesan (see page 53)

extra-virgin olive oil

FUNGI—THE GOOD AND THE BAD:
Never pick a mushroom in the wild if you're not certain whether it's an edible variety. There can be very little difference in appearance between a poisonous and an edible one! Edible mushrooms are healthy and have anti-inflammatory and antiviral properties.

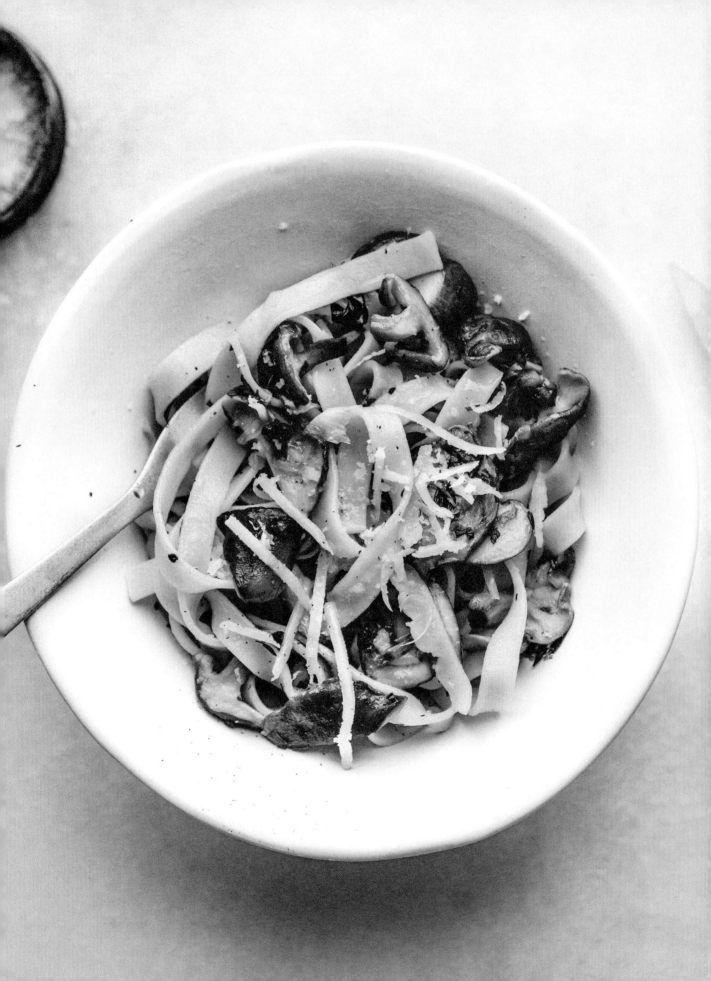

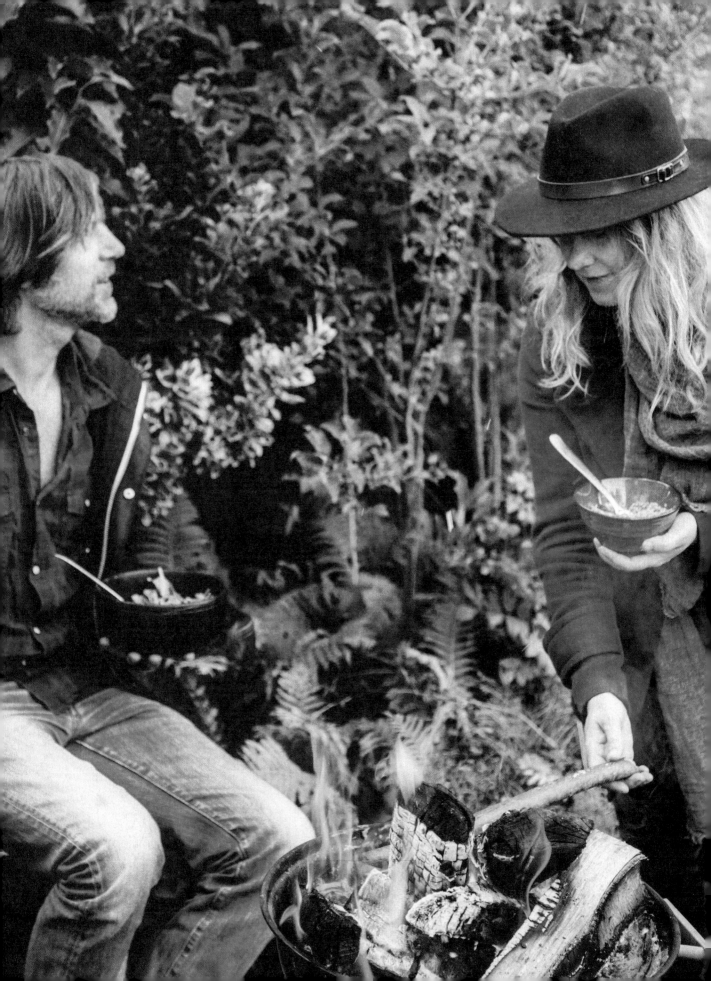

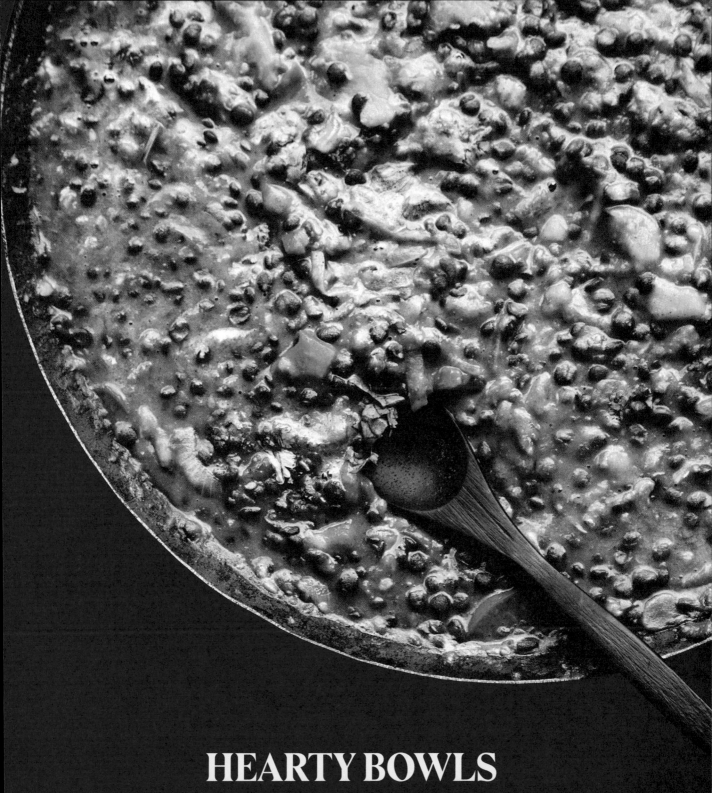

HEARTY BOWLS

We like our food extra-comforting when the weather turns chilly or the skies are gray—a salad just won't do. Instead, it's all about flavorful stews, chilis, and curries! Some of the most delicious food I know belongs in this chapter, in dishes inspired by food from Asia, Morocco, India, France, Britain, and the United States. Truly a taste of the world. Comfort food doesn't have to be heavy, just substantial and nourishing. These recipes are wholesome yet sinfully good.

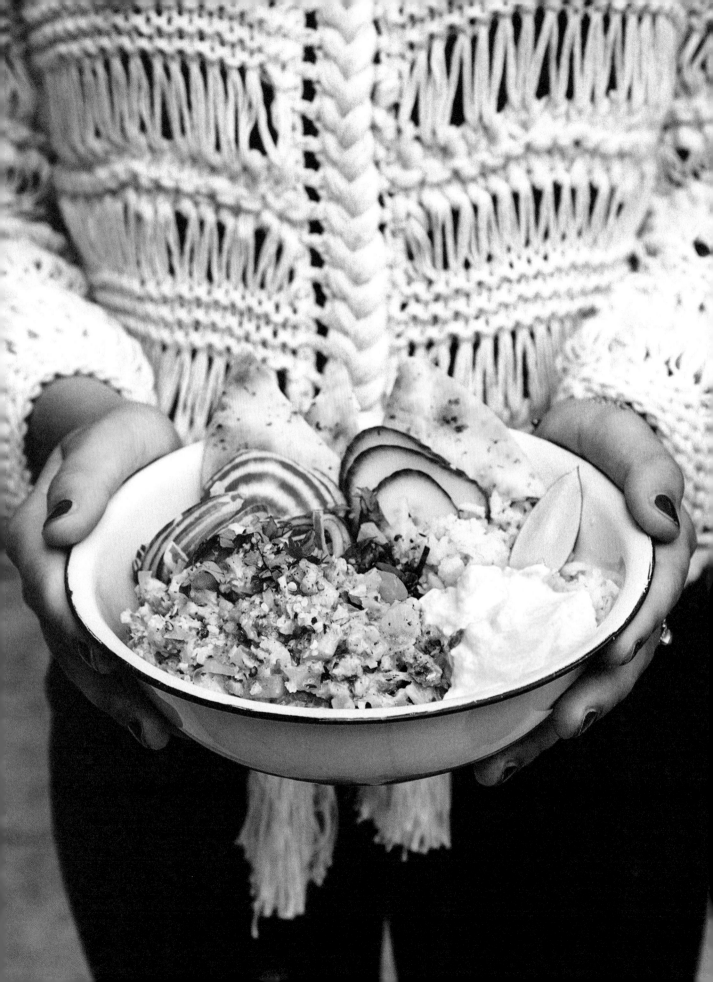

Royal Korma

WITH RAITA AND ONION AND APPLE PICKLE

I fell in love with the sweet and savory wonders of korma during my years living in London. The Bangladeshi curry houses around Brick Lane serve classic anglicized Indian dishes that are bursting with heavenly flavors. The westernized korma is thick and creamy with lots of cilantro and shredded or desiccated coconut. Similar kormas are served in Kerala, in the south of India, where coconut palms grow in abundance. I find these sauces irresistible! A depth of flavor is released by toasting the spices, coconut, and nuts. In India, a very fine korma is called *Shahi korma*. Shahi means royal and, of course, this korma is nothing less than Shahi.

Heat a large skillet over medium-high heat, add 2 tablespoons ghee, and cook the carrots/parsnips and crumbled cauliflower for 5 minutes. Sprinkle with a little salt, remove from the heat, and set aside.

Next make the spice paste by roughly processing all the ingredients. Heat a small skillet over medium-low heat and toast the spice mix until fragrant, 1 to 2 minutes. Remove from the heat and work the mix into a paste using a mortar and pestle (or a food processor).

Heat a large skillet over medium-low heat. Add the remaining ghee and cook the onions for 5 to 8 minutes. Add the korma spice paste and stir for another 1 to 2 minutes. Add the coconut milk, lemon juice, and coconut sugar. Mix well. Finally, add the cauliflower and carrots/parsnips to the pan and let the sauce simmer over low heat for 5 minutes.

Mix the raita ingredients into a smooth sauce. Combine the pickle ingredients. Serve the korma with the raita, pickle, rice, naan, and cilantro.

VE *Use coconut oil instead of ghee.*
For the raita, use coconut yogurt.
GF *Serve without naan bread.*

INDIAN FOOD! *Indian food is a very good choice for vegetarians and vegans. India has a long history of eating plant-based foods and two-thirds of India's population are vegetarians. There's a wealth of flavor in Indian cooking and for those who are skeptical about vegetarian food, show them the light by serving this vibrant dish.*

SERVES 3 TO 4
4 tablespoons ghee or coconut oil
  and more if needed
4 carrots or parsnips, diced small
1 head cauliflower, chopped into
  a crumble
3 red onions, chopped
2 14 oz. cans coconut cream or milk
juice of 1 lemon or lime
3 tablespoons coconut sugar
salt and pepper

KORMA SPICE PASTE
4–5 garlic cloves, finely chopped to
  a paste with 1 teaspoon salt
2 green chile peppers, seeded and
  finely chopped
handful of fresh cilantro, chopped
1 tablespoon freshly grated ginger
3 handfuls of desiccated coconut
2 handfuls of toasted almonds
1 tablespoon tomato paste
1 teaspoon ground turmeric
1 teaspoon ground coriander
½ teaspoon ground cardamom
1 tablespoon ground cumin
½ teaspoon ground cinnamon
pinch of black pepper

RAITA
1 cup yogurt of your choice
¼ cup finely chopped cucumber
splash of apple cider vinegar
handful of mint leaves, finely
  chopped

ONION AND APPLE PICKLE
1 red onion, finely sliced
1 sweet apple, quartered, cored,
  and finely sliced
3 tablespoons apple cider vinegar
1 tablespoon chopped cilantro
few thin slices of chioggia beet
  (optional)

TO SERVE
cooked brown rice, naan bread,
  fresh cilantro

North African Eggplant Stew

EGGPLANT AND SWEET POTATO STEW WITH RAS EL HANOUT

North African stews are full of energizing spices. This recipe is inspired by Moroccan tagines, using ras el hanout for a defining taste. Ras el hanout is usually the finest spice mix in Moroccan spice shops, not a hot spice mix but a comforting one, with cinnamon and cardamom and sometimes rose petals. It's a seductive flavor that Moroccans believe to be an aphrodisiac. This is not a heavy stew, it's a perfect all-year-round dish and works as a summer dinner with its fresh and light flavor.

Heat a large saucepan over medium-high heat and add a drizzle of olive oil. Cook the onion and garlic until the onion is translucent. Add the ras el hanout, cinnamon, and salt, and stir with the onions for 1 to 2 minutes. Add the eggplant, pepper, and sweet potato and cook, stirring, for 2 to 3 minutes. Add the tomatoes, coconut milk, tahini, harissa, cayenne, raisins, and honey. Cover the pan and allow the stew to simmer over low heat for 15 minutes. Taste and adjust the seasoning with salt and pepper.

Meanwhile, cook the couscous according to the package instructions. Serve the stew with couscous, slivered almonds, and mint leaves.

Tip! Make a variation of this stew using chickpeas instead of eggplant.

VE *Use maple syrup in place of the honey.*
GF *Use buckwheat or millet in place of the couscous.*

SERVES 4
olive oil
2 red onions, finely sliced
3 garlic cloves, finely sliced
1 tablespoon ras el hanout
1 teaspoon cinnamon
1 teaspoon salt
2 eggplants, diced
1 red bell pepper, diced
6 sweet potatoes, peeled and diced
14½ oz. can diced tomatoes
14 oz. can coconut milk
1 tablespoon tahini
1 tablespoon harissa paste
¼ teaspoon cayenne pepper
handful of raisins
1 teaspoon honey
salt and pepper

TO SERVE
1½ cups whole-grain couscous
slivered almonds
fresh mint leaves

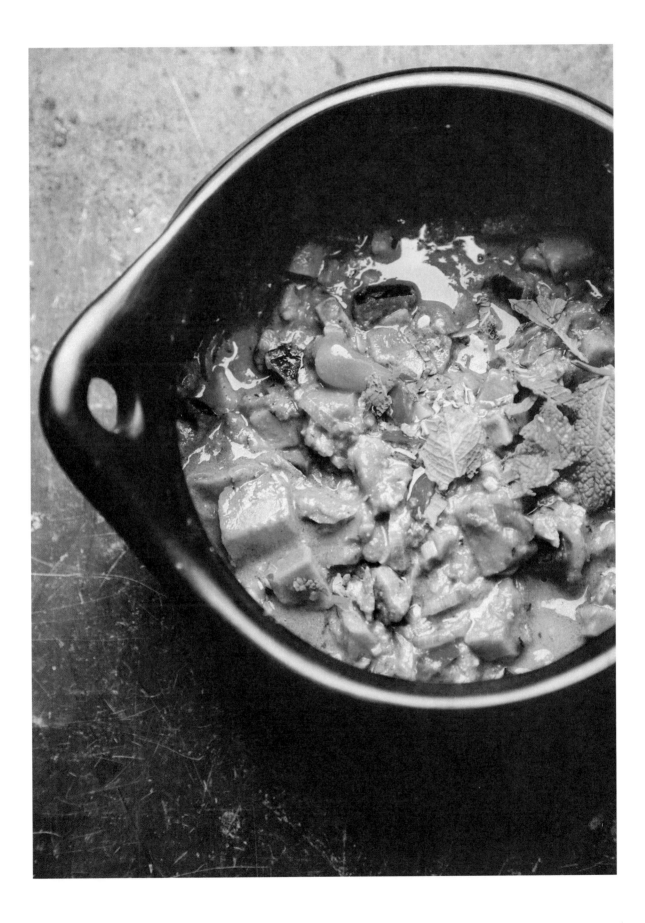

Rendang

INDONESIAN SEITAN AND PARSNIP STEW WITH COCONUT AND KAFFIR LIME

Rendang is a popular Indonesian dish with a generous coconut flavor. Cooking this rendang fills your kitchen with wonderful aromas. This recipe translates the fresh notes of lemongrass, kaffir lime leaves, and coconut into a beautiful stew. The magic in this recipe comes from the underlying flavors of the stew. You can easily substitute filling ingredients such as sweet potato or any other root vegetable for the seitan and parsnip. You could also add chickpeas, beans, or lentils with great results.

Cook the rice according to the package instructions. Drain and set aside. Blend the spice mix into a fine paste in a food processor. Heat a dry wok and toast the coconut until golden brown, stirring with a wooden spoon. Remove from the wok and set aside.

Wipe out the wok and reheat over medium-high heat. Add a drizzle of oil and cook the shallots and parsnips until the shallots are translucent. Add the spice mix and stir. Add the seitan and stir for 2 to 3 minutes. Pour the coconut milk into the wok and bring to a boil. Add the toasted coconut (reserving some for serving), masala curry powder, kaffir lime leaves, garlic paste, lemon juice, maple syrup, soy sauce, and coconut sugar. Let it simmer and reduce for 8 to 10 minutes, stirring with a wooden spoon to avoid burning, until the sauce has thickened. Season with salt and pepper to taste. Remove the lime leaves and serve with toasted coconut, rice, and cilantro.

VE ✓

GF *Use firm tofu instead of seitan. Use gluten-free tamari instead of soy sauce.*

SERVES 4

1½ cups brown rice
1½ cups shredded coconut
coconut oil
6 shallots, finely sliced
2½ cups chopped parsnips, or other root vegetable like carrot, sweet potato, or potato
1¼ lb. seitan
2 x 14 oz. cans coconut milk
1 tablespoon masala curry powder
5 kaffir lime leaves, torn
3 garlic cloves, finely chopped to a paste with 1 teaspoon salt
juice of ½ lemon
3 tablespoons maple syrup
2 tablespoons soy sauce
2 tablespoons coconut sugar
salt and pepper
cilantro leaves, for serving

SPICE MIX

1 teaspoon freshly grated turmeric
1 tablespoon freshly grated galangal
2 tablespoons freshly grated ginger
2 lemongrass stalks, peeled and chopped
5 macadamia nuts (or almonds)
1 fresh bird's eye chile, thinly sliced

INDONESIAN RICE TABLE! *The Dutch culture has a long colonial history with Indonesia and the Dutch are very fond of Indonesian food and restaurants. The "Rijsttafel," meaning rice table, is a much-loved Dutch version of Indonesian cooking. Rendang has a central part on the rice table next to other dishes rich with peanuts, coconut, and lime. Serve this dish followed by a dessert of Nice Cream and Caramel Sauce (see page 178) to experience the flavors of a Dutch Indonesian rice table.*

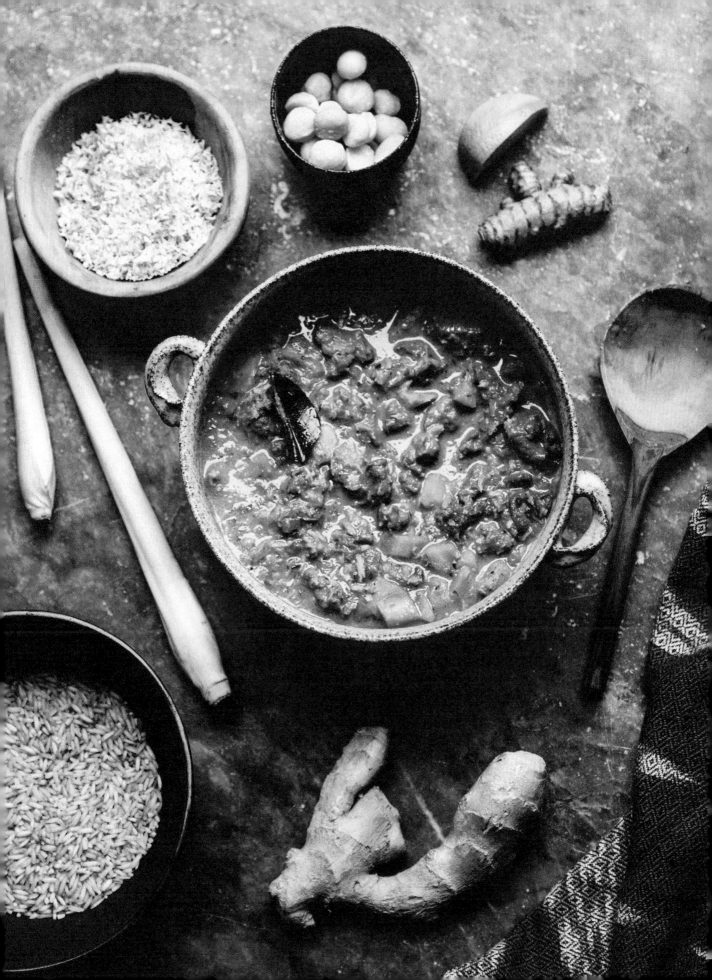

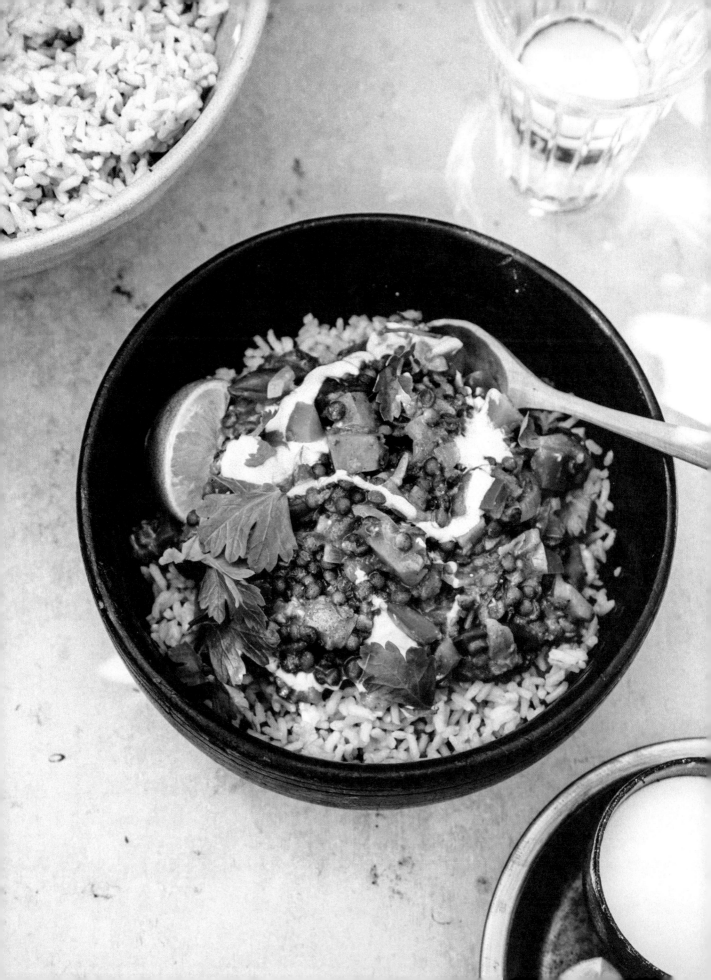

The Loyal Lentil Chili

LENTIL CHILI WITH BUTTERNUT SQUASH, COCONUT MILK, PEPPER, AND LIME

Do you have a dish that never fails you, like a loyal friend, who keeps showing up and impressing you by always being top-notch? I have a few and this lentil chili has been the star of my regular repertoire for years. This is also one of the most frequently prepared and loved recipes from my blog. Lentils can come across as a bit dull sometimes, but this dish is anything but. With flavors that really sing together—earthy cumin and cinnamon, tangy lime and cilantro, hot chile, and garlic—it harmonizes perfectly with sweet butternut squash and chewy lentils. As an alternative to butternut squash you can use cooked pumpkin, eggplant, or any other fleshy vegetable.

Cook the lentils according to the package instructions. Rinse, drain, and set aside. Heat a skillet over medium-high heat. Add the oil and gently cook the shallots until translucent. Add the garlic, spices, red pepper, red chile, and tomatoes. Cook for a few minutes over medium-low heat.

Stir in the lentils, squash, tahini, and honey. Pour in the coconut milk and stir, then simmer over medium-low heat for 5 minutes, adding a little water if needed, and stirring regularly. Add the lime juice and soy sauce, then continue simmering for a few minutes while stirring. Taste and adjust the seasoning with salt and pepper. Remove from the heat.

Mix the ingredients for the yogurt sauce. Make the cucumber salad by combining the shaved cucumber and rice vinegar. Drizzle the chili with extra-virgin olive oil, top with freshly chopped cilantro. Serve with the cool yogurt sauce, cucumber salad, brown rice, lime wedges, and hot sauce.

VE *Use agave syrup instead of honey and vegan yogurt.*

GF *Use gluten-free tamari instead of soy sauce.*

SERVES 4

1 cup Le Puy or black lentils
1 tablespoon coconut or olive oil
5–7 shallots, finely chopped
4 garlic cloves, finely chopped to a
   paste with 1 teaspoon salt
½ tablespoon ground cumin
1 teaspoon ground turmeric
1 teaspoon ground cinnamon
1 teaspoon paprika
1 teaspoon ground coriander
1 red bell pepper, halved, seeded,
   and finely chopped
1–2 red chile peppers, seeded and
   finely chopped
2 tomatoes, finely chopped
1 lb. butternut squash, cooked
   and diced
1 tablespoon tahini
1 tablespoons honey or agave syrup
14 oz. can coconut milk
juice of 1 lime
3 tablespoons soy sauce
salt and pepper

SIMPLE YOGURT SAUCE
1 cup yogurt or vegan yogurt
   (soygurt or coconut yogurt)
1 teaspoon honey or agave syrup
drizzle of extra-virgin olive oil

QUICKEST CUCUMBER SALAD
½ cucumber, shaved into ribbons
¼ cup rice vinegar

TO SERVE
extra-virgin olive oil
fresh cilantro
cooked brown rice or other
   whole grain
lime wedges
hot sauce, like Sriracha

Neatball Masala

NEATBALLS WITH SPICY MASALA SAUCE AND QUICK-PICKLED CARROT RIBBONS

Indian food is the perfect comfort food, adding brightness on gray and cloudy days with a warm spiciness. This sauce can be varied in hotness, so if you want to go easy, use the hot peppers sparingly in the sauce and serve with a chili paste on the side instead, so that each and every eater can add as much as desired. Serve the sauce with neatballs or vegetarian kofta balls.

To make the quick-pickled carrots, mix the carrot ribbons with the water, agave syrup, and rice vinegar. Set aside until ready to serve.

Add the dry spices and lemon juice to a bowl with the ginger, garlic, and chili paste and mix well. Heat a skillet, add a drizzle of oil, and cook the onions over medium heat until they start to caramelize, after a few minutes. Add the ground almonds for the last 2 minutes and toss them with the onions. Remove the onions and almonds from the heat and transfer to the bowl of spices. Using a food processor, blend the ingredients together to form a paste.

Add the spice paste back into the pan with the tomato paste, coconut cream, vegetable broth, soy sauce, and olive oil. Mix well and simmer over low heat for 10 to 15 minutes. Taste and adjust with salt. Serve with rice, neatballs, pickles, and raita and hemp seeds (optional).

Tip! The sauce can be reheated before serving. It will only make it more delicious if it sits so the flavors infuse.

VE *If serving with raita, use vegan yogurt.*
GF *Use firm tofu instead of seitan. Use gluten-free tamari instead of soy sauce.*

SERVES 3 TO 4

QUICK-PICKLED CARROTS
2 carrots, sliced into thin ribbons
$1/4$ cup water
2 tablespoons agave syrup
$1/4$ cup rice vinegar

SPICE PASTE FOR THE SAUCE
$1^{1}/_{2}$ tablespoons garam masala
1 teaspoon ground cardamom
1 teaspoon ground cloves
1 teaspoon ground turmeric
1 tablespoon ground coriander
1 teaspoon ground cumin
1 tablespoon paprika
1 teaspoon salt
juice of $1/2$ lemon
$1^{1}/_{2}$ tablespoons freshly grated ginger
4 garlic cloves, finely chopped to a paste
$1/2$–2 tablespoons chili paste or minced fresh red chile pepper (some like it hot, others not)
coconut or olive oil
2 red onions, chopped
2 tablespoons ground almonds

SAUCE BASE
$1/4$ cup tomato paste
14 oz. can coconut cream
$1^{1}/_{4}$ cup vegetable broth
$1/4$ cup soy sauce
2 tablespoons olive oil, for roasting

SERVE WITH
neatballs (see page 164)
brown rice
raita (see page 133)
sprinkles of hemp seeds

VARIATIONS! *This flavorful sauce can be used as a base for various add-ins. Serve it with roasted cauliflower, chickpeas, lentils, sweet potato, or other root vegetables.*

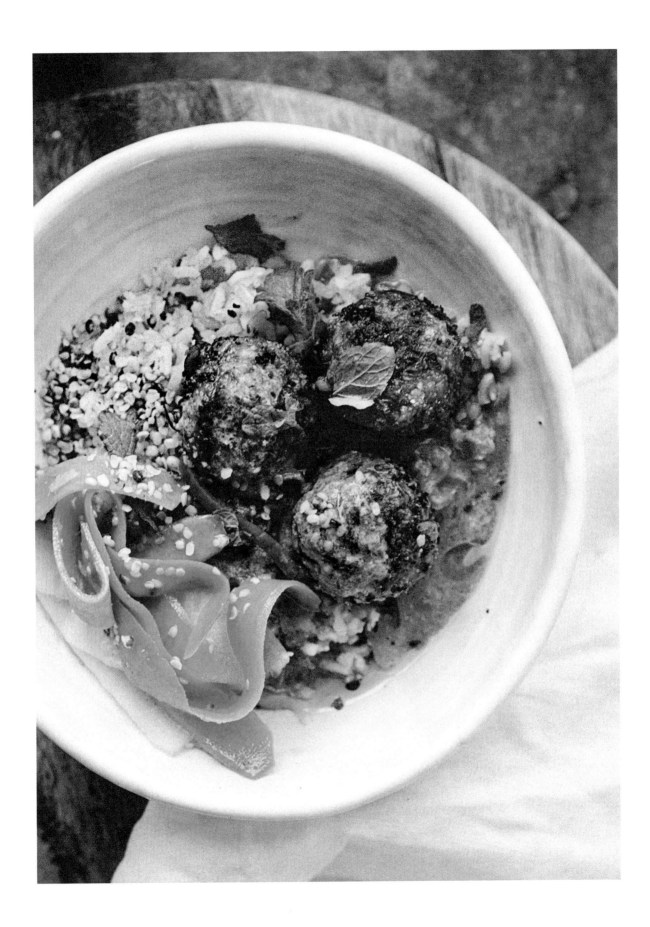

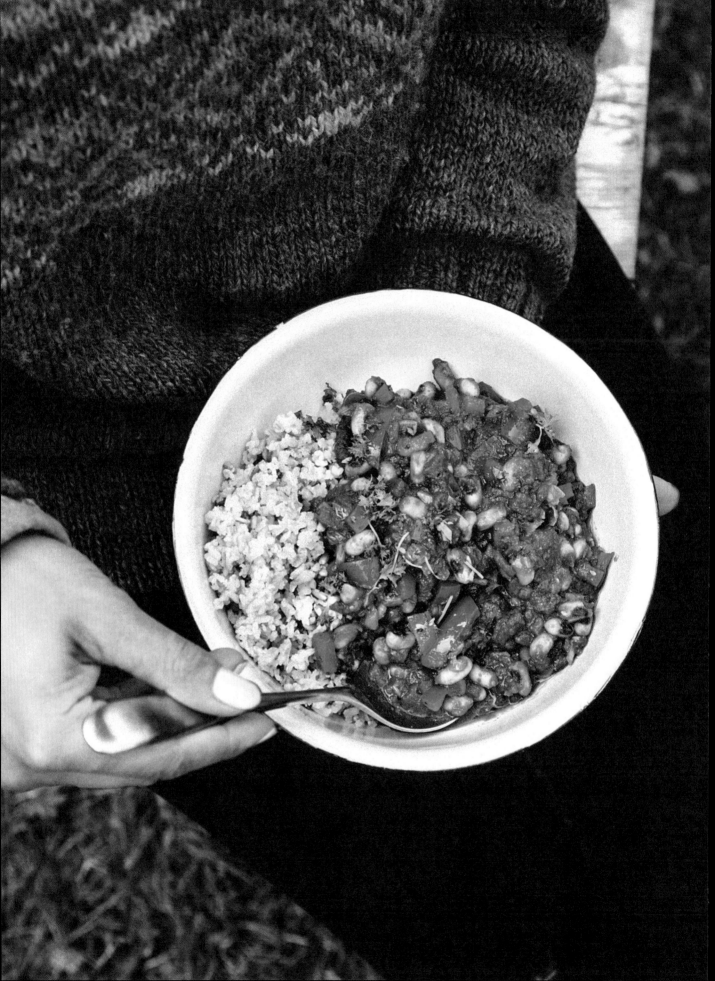

Chili de Frijoles

BEAN STEW WITH RAW CACAO, PEPPERS, AND OREGANO

Chilis are the perfect way to fill us up and this bean dish is popular with people of all ages! For the young ones I use less chili powder, and they like to hear that this chili is flavored with a little cacao—the same ingredient used to make chocolate. The difference between cacao and cocoa is that the former is unroasted, cold-pressed cacao beans. By not roasting the cacao, the high nutritional value stays optimized.

Cacao is a popular ingredient in savory Mexican dishes and it gives an interesting character to this stew. The clean and invigorating heat with the warming spices and herbs make this humble bean stew a comfort super bowl.

Heat a large saucepan over medium-high heat and add a drizzle of olive oil. Cook the onion and garlic until the onion is translucent. Add the red pepper and cook for another 3 to 4 minutes. Add the herbs and spices, except the cacao, and stir with the onion for a minute. Next add the peas and the tomatoes and stir. Simmer and reduce for 5 minutes.

Remove from heat and mix in the raw cacao. Season with salt and pepper to taste and serve with rice, topped with fresh parsley.

VE ✓ GF ✓

SERVES 4
olive oil
2–3 onions, finely chopped
3–4 garlic cloves, finely chopped
2 red bell peppers, finely chopped
$\frac{1}{2}$–1 tablespoon chipotle or ancho chili powder or other chili powder (adjust heat to taste)
$1\frac{1}{2}$ tablespoons dried oregano
1 tablespoon cumin
1 teaspoon paprika
$\frac{1}{2}$ teaspoon ground cinnamon
1 tablespoon brown sugar (or coconut sugar)
2 $14\frac{1}{2}$ oz. cans black-eyed peas
$14\frac{1}{2}$ oz. can diced tomatoes
1 teaspoon raw cacao powder (or cocoa powder)
salt and pepper

TO SERVE
rice
fresh parsley leaves

COFFEE-FLAVORED CHILI: *For a fun twist and variation, add ¾ cup freshly brewed coffee and let the chili reduce for a few minutes longer. It gives the chili an interesting extra flavor dimension. The taste of coffee is more suitable for grown-up eaters than children.*

Back to the Roots

BROCCOLI MASH, ROASTED VEGGIES, AND SPROUTS WITH A CARROT MISO SAUCE

This recipe is inspired by the idea of cooking without a recipe! I frequently fall in love with ingredients not on my shopping list and come home with bags of the most vibrant-looking food I can find, rather than the food I had planned. This often results in an alternative tapas-style dinner. I like to enjoy really fresh and beautiful produce by cooking ingredients separately for maximum flavor and freshness. Steaming is one of the best ways to keep nutrition and flavor in broccoli, whereas kale releases its nutritional power and flavor best when the cellulose structure is broken down through stir-frying. By cooking the main ingredients differently you get a variety of textures and flavors to enjoy. A good cold sauce ties everything together beautifully.

Preheat the oven to 400°F and line a baking sheet with parchment. Put the sweet potato, onion, and pumpkin seeds on the lined baking sheet and drizzle with the olive oil. Sprinkle with paprika, thyme, cumin seeds, and salt. Roast for 35 minutes. Turn the roasting veggies halfway through and keep an eye on them to make sure they don't burn.

Meanwhile, make the broccoli mash. Steam the broccoli florets for 4 minutes. Transfer to a food processor with 2 tablespoons of extra-virgin olive oil and a good pinch of salt, tahini, garlic, lemon juice, and hemp seeds. Blend to a chunky mash, adding more olive oil if needed. Keep warm in the oven until ready to serve.

Remove the thick stalks from the kale and tear the leaves into pieces. Heat a skillet with a drizzle of olive oil and cook the kale over medium-high heat, stirring, for 3 to 4 minutes. Add a drizzle of soy sauce, lemon juice, crushed garlic clove, and sesame seeds. Sprinkle with nutritional yeast or Parmesan and remove from the heat.

Blend the ingredients for the sauce, adding enough water to achieve the required consistency.

Drizzle the roasted veggies and kale with the sauce and serve with fresh micro sprouts, spinach, or herbs tossed with a little toasted sesame oil and cider vinegar.

VE *Use nutritional yeast instead of Parmesan.*

GF *Use gluten-free tamari instead of soy sauce.*

SERVES 4

ROASTED VEGGIES
5 sweet potatoes, peeled and
   cut into chunks
2 red onions, quartered
¼ cup pumpkin seeds
olive oil
1 teaspoon paprika
1 teaspoon fresh thyme
1 teaspoon cumin seeds
salt

BROCCOLI MASH
2 lbs. broccoli florets
3 tablespoons extra-virgin olive oil
3 tablespoons tahini
1 garlic clove
juice of ½ lemon
2 handfuls of hemp seeds

SAUTÉED KALE
big bunch of kale
olive oil
soy sauce
good squeeze of lemon juice
1 garlic clove, crushed
handful of toasted sesame seeds
2 tablespoons nutritional yeast
   or Parmesan

MISO, TAHINI, CARROT SAUCE
1 carrot, finely grated
1 tablespoon miso paste
1 tablespoon tahini
juice of ½ lemon
2 tablespoons extra-virgin olive oil
1 garlic clove, finely chopped
   to a paste

CLEAN SALAD
fresh micro sprouts
spinach
fresh herbs
toasted sesame oil
apple cider vinegar

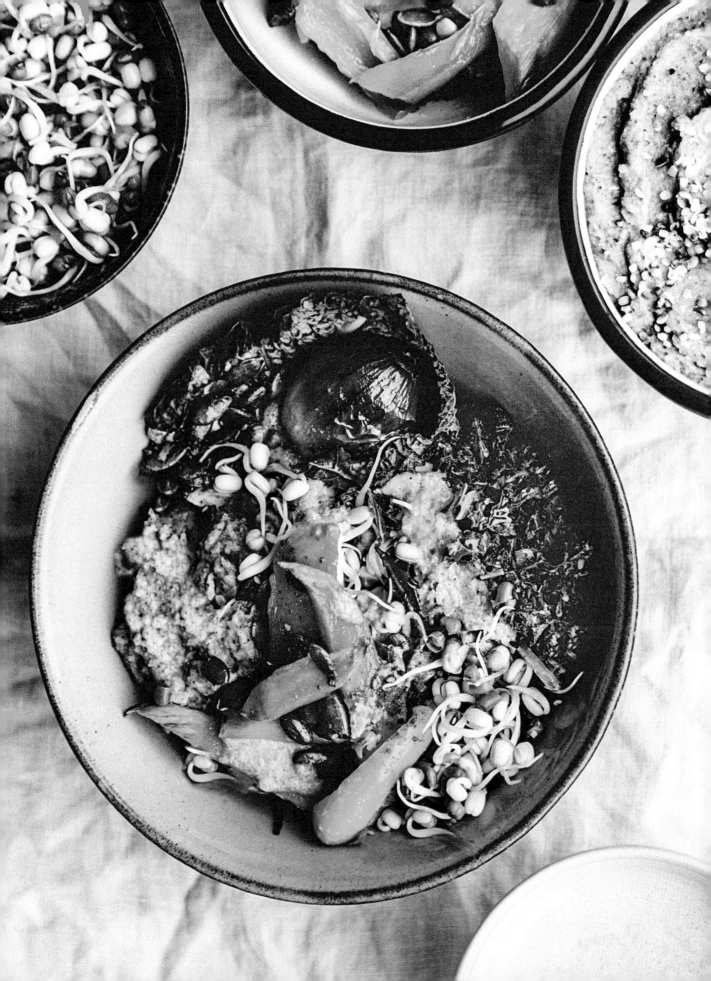

Pulled Jackfruit

FAUX PULLED PORK WITH CREAMY COLESLAW AND ROOT WEDGES

Liquid smoke adds a smoky touch to this recipe inspired by barbecue flavors. The texture of jackfruit makes it perfect to sauté and cover with homemade barbecue sauce for a delicious faux pulled-pork meal. This mouthwatering, plant-based riff on Southern-style barbecue will satisfy your cravings. Though this bowl has a sinful appearance, it's actually light, guilt-free, and totally wholesome. Buy jackfruit in water (not in brine) online or from Asian food stores and well-stocked supermarkets.

First roast the wedges. Preheat the oven to 400°F and line a baking sheet with parchment. Arrange the sweet potatoes on the baking sheet, toss with a drizzle of olive oil, and sprinkle with salt. Roast for 25 minutes or until the sweet potato is soft. Turn the baking sheet around after 15 minutes and keep an eye on the wedges during the last 10 minutes as you don't want them to burn.

Meanwhile, make the coleslaw. Put the carrot, apple, and shredded cabbage in a large bowl. Whisk olive oil, mayonnaise, apple cider, and mustard in a small bowl, then mix with the cabbage. Season with salt and pepper to taste.

Mix the barbecue sauce ingredients in a bowl and set aside. Drain the jackfruit. Heat a skillet over medium-high heat, add a drizzle of olive oil and sauté the shallots until translucent. Add another drizzle of olive oil and the jackfruit, garlic paste, and mushrooms and sauté for 2 more minutes. Cover the jackfruit in vegetable broth and let it simmer, covered, over medium-low heat until the jackfruit starts breaking into threads, about 10 minutes. Add the barbecue sauce and let it all simmer and reduce for 10 to 12 minutes over medium-low heat while stirring.

Remove from the heat and swirl in some extra-virgin olive oil. Stir in the liquid smoke. Taste and adjust the seasoning with salt and pepper. Serve with the sweet potato wedges, coleslaw, and additional hot sauce.

VE *Use Vegenaise instead of mayonnaise.*
Replace honey with agave syrup.

GF *Use gluten-free tamari instead*
of soy sauce.

SMOKE IN A BOTTLE: *Liquid smoke might sound like a magical potion, but it's actually smoke that's been collected from burning wood. It's used in gastronomy and by vegans for flavor enhancement. Adding liquid smoke adds a beautiful smoky flavor that our human taste buds find irresistible. Find it online and in culinary shops that sell vegan products.*

SERVES 2

3 sweet potatoes, peeled and
    cut into wedges
olive oil
14½ oz. can green jackfruit
2 shallots, finely sliced
2 garlic cloves, finely chopped to a
    paste with 1 teaspoon salt
½ lb. shiitake mushrooms, chopped
1¼ cup vegetable broth
2 teaspoons liquid smoke (optional)
salt and pepper

COLESLAW

2 carrots, julienned
1 sweet firm apple, quartered,
    cored, and thinly sliced
2 cups finely shredded white
    cabbage leaves
2 tablespoons extra-virgin olive oil
¼ cup mayonnaise or Vegenaise
2 tablespoons apple cider vinegar
1 tablespoon mustard
salt and pepper

BARBECUE SAUCE

2 tablespoons palm sugar
1 teaspoon Dijon mustard
1 teaspoon chili sauce (Sriracha
    or similar)
few grinds of black pepper
¾ teaspoon salt
2 teaspoons paprika
1 teaspoon tamarind paste
2 tablespoons soy sauce
1 teaspoon honey
1 teaspoon fennel seeds, ground
1 teaspoon tomato ketchup
⅔ cup water

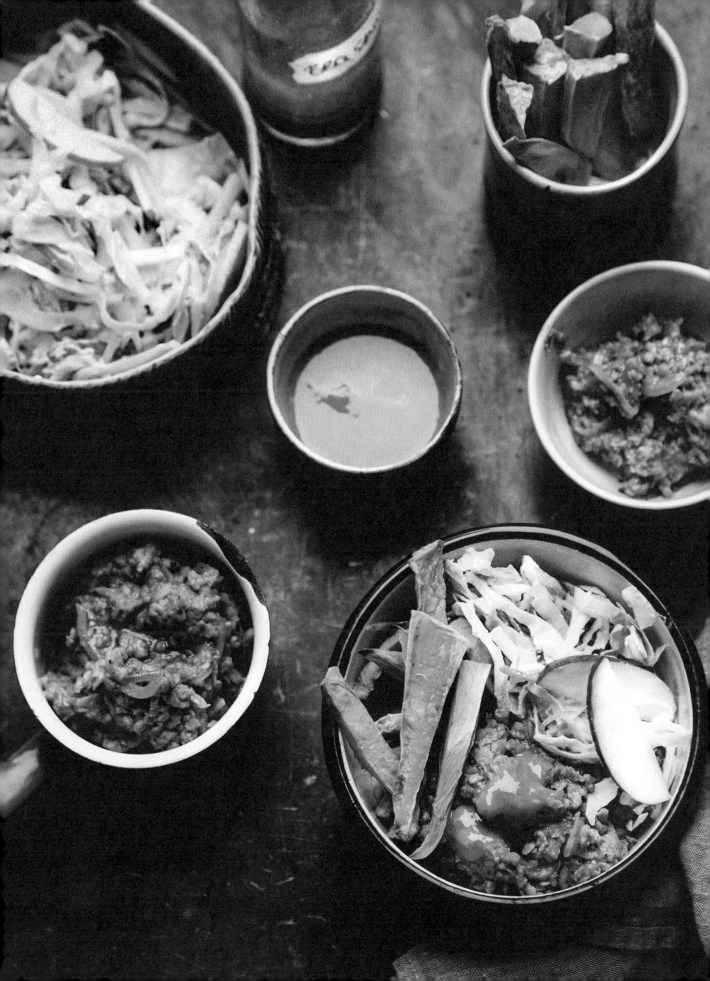

Chanterelle Risotto

BROWN RICE RISOTTO WITH TARRAGON SAUTÉED MUSHROOMS

Risotto is both filling and comforting, and makes a lovely base for sautéed mushrooms. This autumn classic can be made with various grains or quinoa, just adjust the simmering time accordingly. Use whole-grain brown rice for a health boost and soak your rice overnight to reduce the cooking time. You could also top with roasted vegetables instead of chanterelles.

Heat a large skillet over medium-high heat and add a drizzle of olive oil. Cook the shallots and garlic until the shallots are translucent. Add the rice and cook for another 2 minutes. Add the wine, then the broth ladle by ladle. Simmer over medium-low heat for 20 to 25 minutes while stirring to avoid burning.

Remove from the heat and mix in the Parmesan. Season with salt and pepper to taste. Heat a skillet and add a drizzle of olive oil or a tablespoon of butter. Cook the chanterelles and tarragon over medium-high heat until golden and fragrant. Season to taste. Serve with the risotto and baby spinach.

VE *Use rawmesan instead of Parmesan and olive oil instead of butter.*

GF ✓

SERVES 2

olive oil
2 shallots, finely chopped
1 garlic clove, finely chopped
  to a paste
1 cup brown rice or brown arborio
  rice, soaked overnight
1 cup white wine
4 cups vegetable broth
1½ cups Parmesan or rawmesan
  (see page 53)
salt and pepper
olive oil or butter
¾ lb. chanterelles or mushrooms
  of your choice
1 tablespoon tarragon leaves,
  chopped
bunch of baby spinach

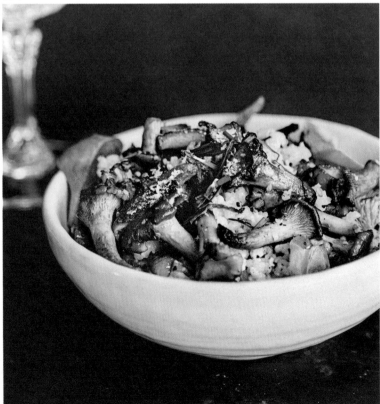

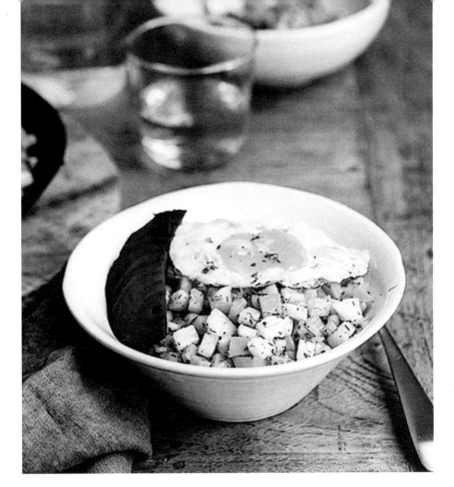

Pyttipanna

HERBED CELERY ROOT, SWEET POTATO, AND HALLOUMI HASH WITH PICKLED BEETS

Pyttipanna means "this and that in a pan" in Swedish, and it's a typical fridge clear-out hash that can be made with various ingredients. Serving pyttipanna is a good way to introduce children to the beautiful flavors of more intimidating root vegetables like celeriac.

To pickle the beets, place the slices in a small bowl with the water, vinegar, and agave syrup and set aside.

Clean and peel the root vegetables and cut into equally sized small cubes (½ to 1 inch). Heat a skillet over medium-high heat and add a tablespoon of butter. Cook the onion until translucent, about 4 to 5 minutes, then add the diced root vegetables and herbs. Cook for 7 to 8 minutes while stirring. Add the halloumi and cook 5 minutes more, or until the root vegetables are soft. Taste and season with salt and pepper.

Divide the pyttipanna between three or four serving bowls and top with a fried sunny-side-up egg, the pickled beets, and some fresh dill.

VE *Use coconut oil instead of butter and omit the egg.*

GF ✓

SERVES 3 TO 4
1–2 lbs. mixed root vegetables—
   celeriac, parsnip, carrot
1 tablespoon butter, ghee, or
   coconut oil
2 onions, finely chopped
1 tablespoon fresh thyme
1 teaspoon chopped rosemary
1 tablespoon dill fronds
¾ lb. halloumi, diced
salt and pepper

PICKLED BEETS
1 beet, trimmed and very
   finely sliced
½ cup water
2 tablespoons red wine vinegar
3 tablespoons agave syrup

TO SERVE
1 fried egg per serving
fresh dill

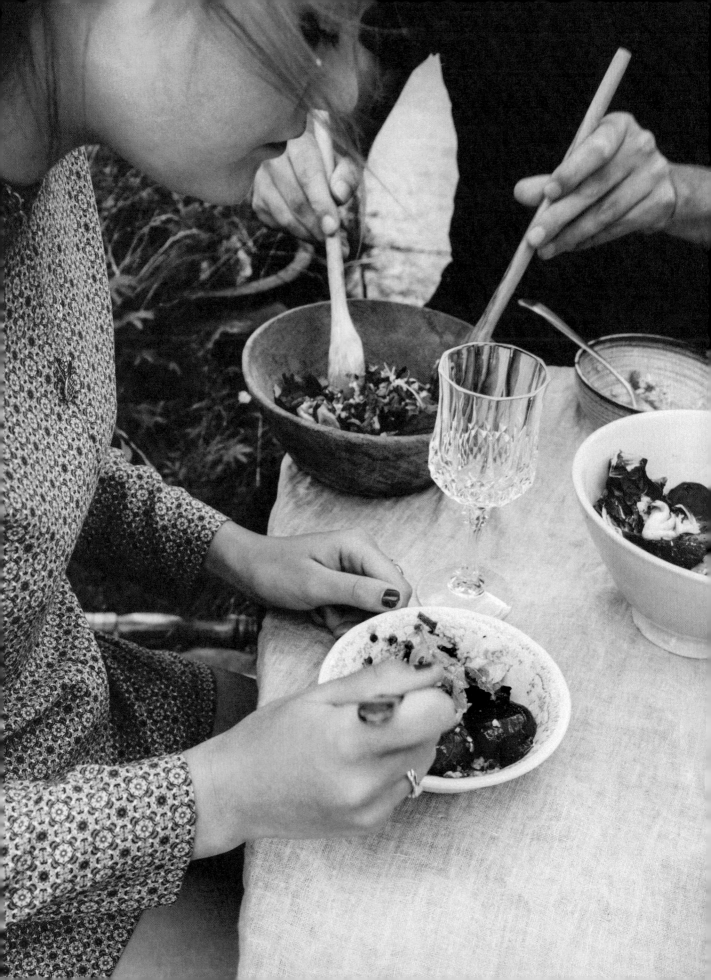

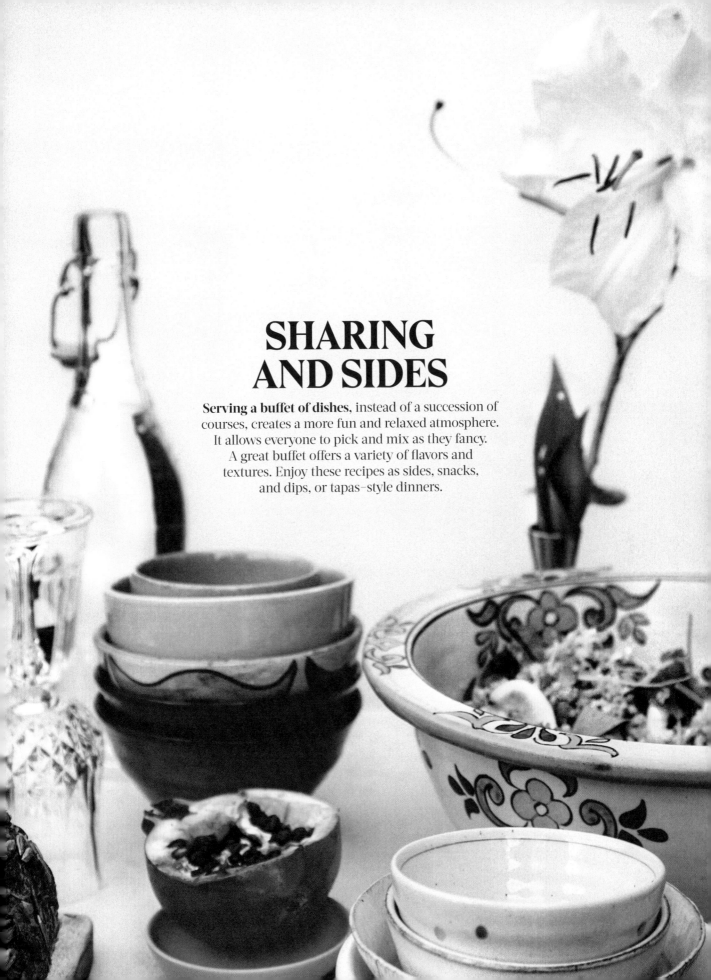

SHARING
AND SIDES

Serving a buffet of dishes, instead of a succession of
courses, creates a more fun and relaxed atmosphere.
It allows everyone to pick and mix as they fancy.
A great buffet offers a variety of flavors and
textures. Enjoy these recipes as sides, snacks,
and dips, or tapas-style dinners.

Tabbouleh with Feta and Pomegranate

HERBED MILLET WITH POMEGRANATE AND FETA

To achieve the necessary fresh tanginess of the best tabbouleh, you need to use the best-quality herbs, tomatoes, and lemon. They will shine in this dish. This tabbouleh is made with fluffy millet instead of the traditional bulgur wheat used in the Middle East. The millet is toasted before cooking, which adds a delicious nutty flavor. When I make tabbouleh I usually add parsley, cilantro, and mint in equal parts rather than just using lots of parsley. Another tweak is the addition of pomegranate seeds. They're sweet and tangy and a perfect counterpart to the salty feta. Tabbouleh is a great side dish, a perfect companion to grilled vegetables and halloumi, or anywhere rice and couscous would be served. You can use any type of grain for this recipe—whole-grain couscous and freekeh are delicious, too—but adjust the cooking time accordingly.

Heat a saucepan and dry-toast the millet over medium heat until golden, about 3 minutes, watching closely so it doesn't burn. Carefully add the water to the hot pan, along with a pinch of salt and stir. Bring to a boil, then turn down the heat and simmer for 15 minutes. Remove from the heat and let it rest, covered. Use a sieve to sift the ground spices into the millet while fluffing with a fork.

Add the diced tomatoes to a bowl and mix with the lemon juice, garlic, olive oil, and honey. Just before serving, mix the seasoned tomatoes, herbs, pomegranate seeds, scallions, and feta in a big bowl with the millet. Sprinkle with salt to taste. Divide the tabbouleh into serving bowls.

VE *Omit the feta. Substitute agave or maple*
syrup for honey.

GF ✓

SERVES 4

1 cup millet

3 cups water

½ teaspoon each of the following
  ground spices: cinnamon,
  coriander, fenugreek

¼ teaspoon black pepper

4–6 ripe, best-quality tomatoes,
  diced small

juice of 1 lemon

1 garlic clove, finely chopped
  to a paste

2 tablespoons extra-virgin olive oil

1 teaspoon honey or agave syrup

big bunch of herbs (parsley,
  cilantro, and mint), finely
  chopped

seeds from 1 pomegranate

4–5 scallions, finely sliced

1–2 cups feta, crumbled

salt

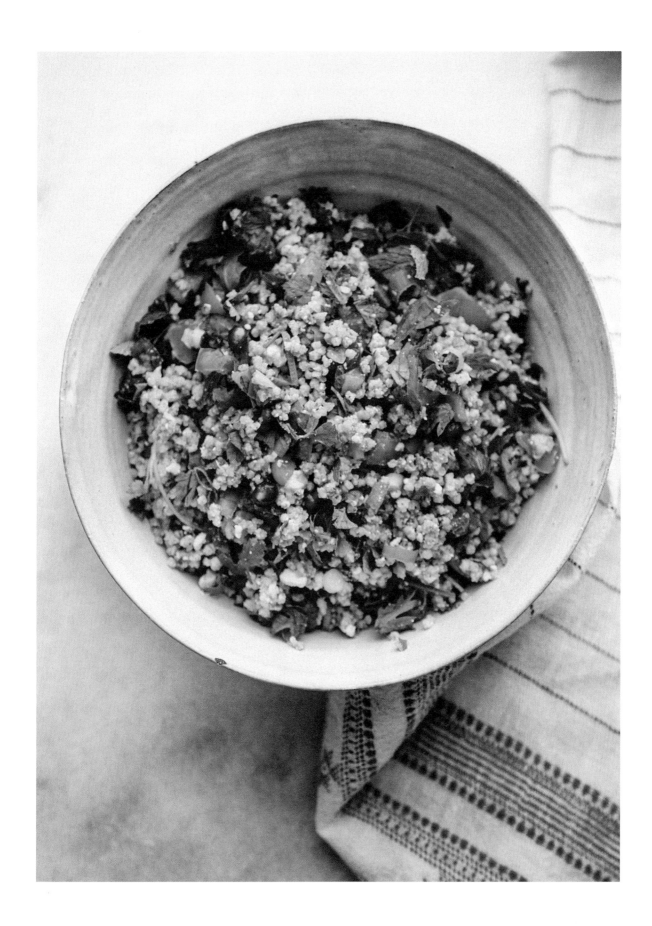

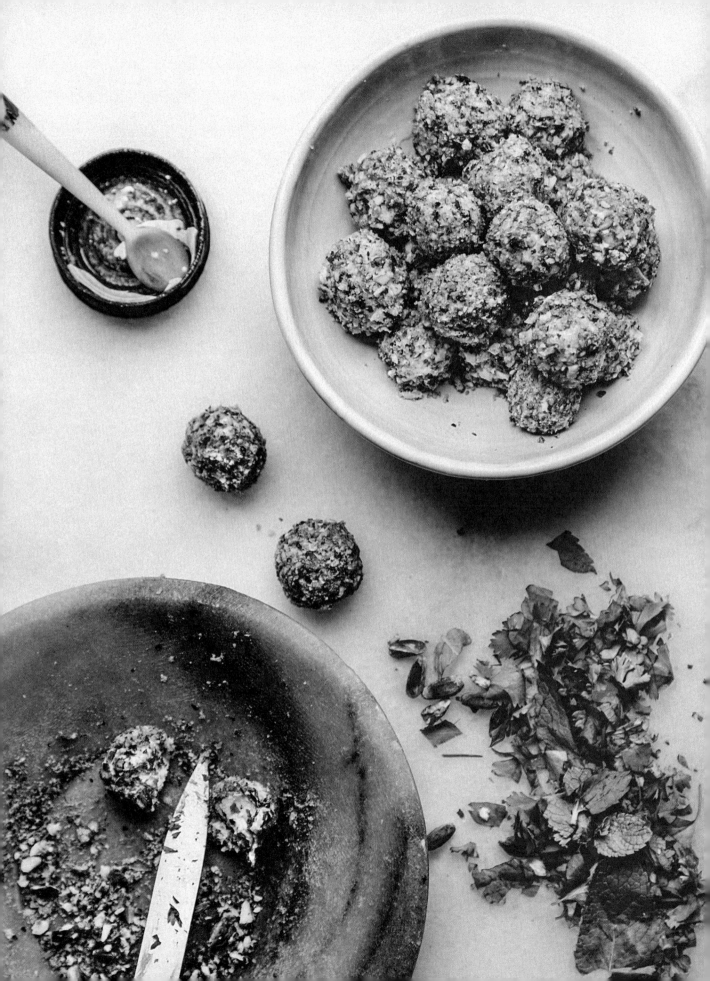

Chèvre Balls

GOAT CHEESE ROLLED IN PISTACHIO

Chèvre balls are the perfect party food. Rolling goat cheese in nuts and then drizzling the herb-flavored balls with honey results in pure deliciousness. Serve as an appetizer or side dish, or add them to a clean green salad. They are best just after they've been made, so serve immediately.

Mix the goat cheese with the herbs and season with salt and pepper to taste. Roll the herbed cheese into small balls with your hands, then roll lightly in the crushed pistachios. Sprinkle with salt and top with a little parsley. Serve as a snack or add to a salad bowl.

Alternative to goat cheese: To make a vegan version of the cheese ball, make your own vegan nut cheese. Process the ingredients for the nut cheese in a food processor until smooth. Let the cashew cheese sit in the fridge, covered, for 1 hour before rolling and coating with pistachios. Serve as you would the chèvre balls.

VE *Use the nut cheese instead of goat cheese. Use agave or maple syrup instead of honey.*

GF ✓

SERVES 8 TO 10 AS A SIDE DISH
$1\frac{1}{2}$ pounds soft goat cheese
bunch of fresh delicate herbs, like
    basil, thyme, and parsley, finely
    chopped
$1\frac{1}{2}$ cups pistachios, finely crushed
clear honey
parsley
salt and pepper

NUT CHEESE
    (alternative to goat cheese)
4 cups raw cashews, soaked
    overnight, then drained
2 tablespoons nutritional yeast
1 garlic clove
juice of 1 lemon

NUT CHEESE! *Nut cheeses are not just for vegans. They're an option for dairy intolerant eaters and a great way to consume less animal protein. Use the basic nut cheese in this recipe with different herbs and spices for a variety of flavors. Nut cheese makes great spreads and creamy dips and sauces.*

Pumpkin Hummus with Mushrooms and Pickled Eggs

BUTTERNUT SQUASH HUMMUS WITH GARLICKY CREMINI MUSHROOMS AND EGGS

This hummus has an extra sweet and silken quality because it contains butternut squash. Topping it with garlicky mushrooms and eggs creates a beautiful harmony of flavors and textures. This dish can be shared as part of a buffet. You can also serve it with yogurt and crudités.

For the pickled eggs, put the beet halves in a pan, cover with water, and simmer for 40 minutes. Let the beet cool in its juices. Place the peeled eggs in a large jar and pour in the apple cider vinegar. Add the sugar, onion, and oregano. Fill the jar with the beet halves and their cooking water. Cover and refrigerate for at least one hour—preferably overnight—to give a more intense color and pickled flavor.

Blend the hummus ingredients to a smooth consistency, adding the water gradually until you reach your desired thickness.

Heat a skillet over medium-high heat. Add a drizzle of olive oil and the garlic and stir for 20 to 30 seconds. Add the mushrooms and tarragon and cook until golden brown and fragrant, about 4 to 5 minutes. Season with salt and pepper to taste.

Serve the hummus with a drizzle of extra-virgin olive oil, mushrooms, and the pickled eggs sliced in half. Top with parsley, sumac, a drizzle of extra-virgin olive oil, and some bread for scooping up the hummus.

VE *Instead of eggs, pickle cubes of firm tofu for 20 minutes in the beet marinade. Drain well before serving.*
GF *Serve with gluten-free bread.*

SERVES 4 TO 6 AS A SIDE DISH

PICKLED EGGS
1 red beet, halved
8 medium eggs, cooked for 7 minutes, cooled, and peeled
³/₄ cup apple cider vinegar
1 teaspoon sugar
1 red onion, sliced into thin rounds
1 teaspoon fresh oregano

HUMMUS
2 14¹/₂-oz. cans chickpeas, drained and rinsed
4 garlic cloves, finely chopped to a paste
¹/₂ cup tahini
1 teaspoon salt
zest and juice of 1 lemon
³/₄ lb. cooked butternut squash or pumpkin, chopped
¹/₂ cup ice-cold water, plus extra if needed
extra-virgin olive oil

MUSHROOMS
olive oil
1 garlic clove, finely chopped to a paste
¹/₂ lb. cremini or portobello mushrooms, cleaned and sliced
1 tablespoon tarragon leaves
salt and pepper

TO SERVE
parsley
sumac
extra-virgin olive oil
bread

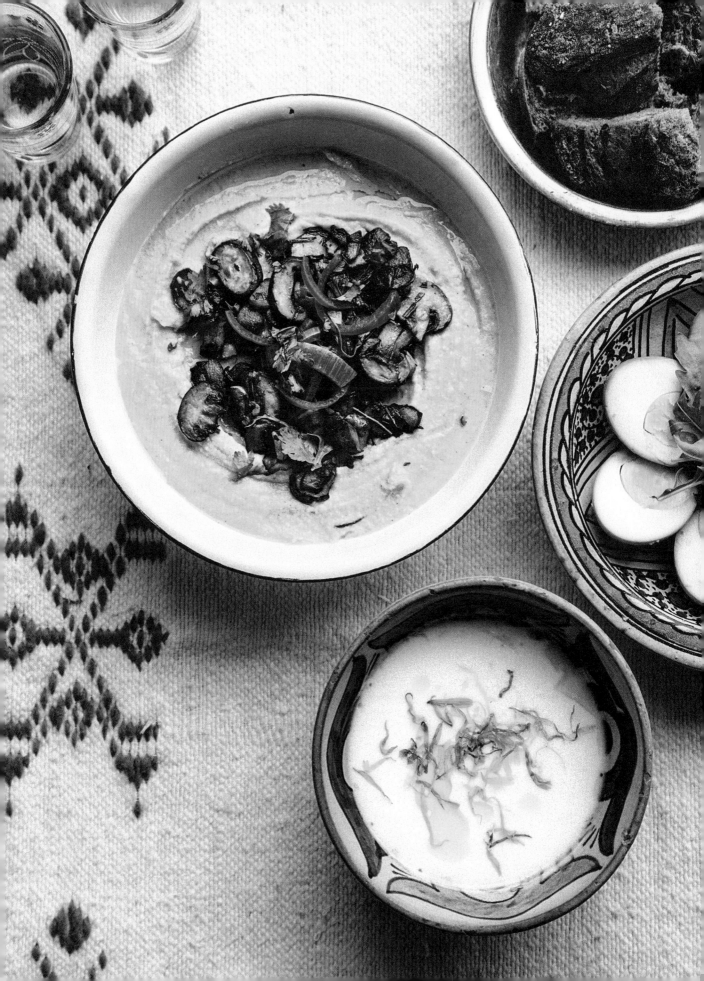

Butternut Squash Cheese Fondue

CRUDITÉS WITH BUTTERNUT SQUASH CHEESE DIP

Cheese fondue was immensely popular in the 1970s and '80s, but while its trendiness waned in the rest of the world, in Holland it was featured on café menus for decades. Lately it has made a comeback, especially with the original plant-based cheese sauces that a new generation of fondue lovers are dipping into. Butternut squash with paprika, garlic, and nutritional yeast makes a delicious cheesy sauce. It's so easy to make and you can vary the crudités according to the season.

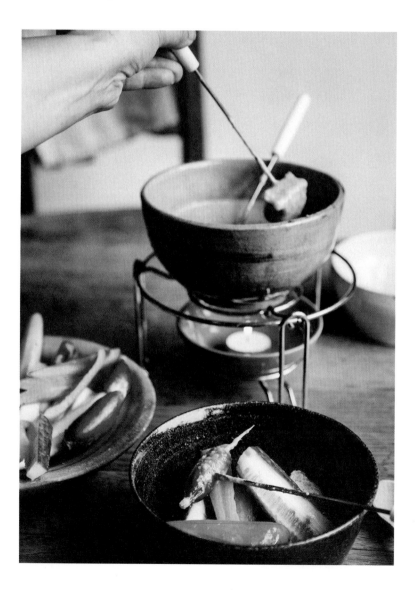

SERVES 6 TO 8 AS A SIDE DISH

2–3 lbs. mixed raw vegetables, such as radishes, cucumber, cauliflower florets, bell peppers, cherry tomatoes

BUTTERNUT SQUASH SAUCE

2 lbs. butternut squash, peeled, seeded, and cut into small wedges
3 tablespoons olive oil
handful of sage leaves, chopped
14 oz. can coconut milk
$\frac{1}{3}$ cup nutritional yeast
1 tablespoon paprika
1 teaspoon Dijon mustard
juice of 2 lemons
4 garlic cloves, crushed
salt and pepper

Preheat the oven to 400°F. Prepare the crudités by cleaning and cutting the vegetables to the desired size. Put the butternut squash wedges on a baking sheet lined with parchment. Drizzle with an even layer of olive oil and sprinkle with salt and sage. Roast for 25 to 30 minutes and remove from the oven. Blend the squash with the rest of the sauce ingredients in a food processor, adding enough water to achieve the desired consistency. Serve with the crudités. You can also dip in bread, of course.

If you don't own a fondue set that will keep the butternut cheese warm while dipping, heat the sauce and serve it hot in a bowl.

VE ✓ GF ✓

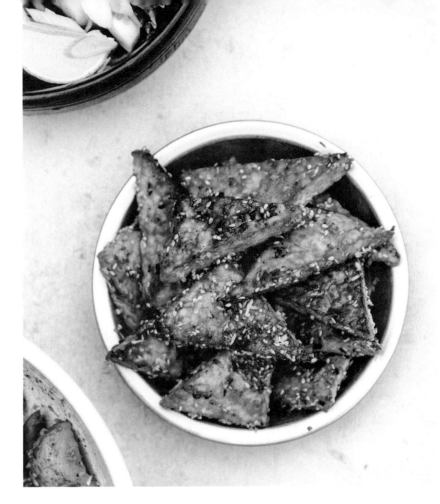

Tempeh Steaks

CHILE-MARINATED TEMPEH WITH CRISPY COCONUT AND SESAME CRUST

These small tempeh steaks, with their distinctive Asian flavor, make delicious little bites. Coated with chile and soy sauce, they accompany noodles, rice, or salad perfectly, and are a regular in my weekday meals. With more bite and structure than seitan and tofu, tempeh makes a great plant-based replacement for meat. These steaks are particularly versatile and will be a satisfying addition to your lunch bowls or even as your "meat" on a grill. If you like to prep ahead, keep the marinated tempeh in the fridge for a maximum of 2 days before cooking. It's best eaten immediately after frying, but will keep for another day in the fridge.

Mix the marinade ingredients in a sealable plastic bag. Toss the tempeh into the marinade and refrigerate for 30 minutes.

Mix the coconut, sesame seeds, and palm sugar in a bowl. Heat a skillet over medium-high heat and melt the coconut oil. Remove the tempeh triangles from the marinade and coat them with the coconut mixture. Fry for 3 to 4 minutes on each side, working in batches, and keeping them warm in a low oven while you fry the rest. Serve with fresh cilantro.

VE ✓

GF *Use gluten-free tamari instead of soy sauce.*

SERVES 6 AS A SIDE DISH

1½ lbs. tempeh, cut into triangles about ¼-inch thick
2 cups shredded coconut
⅓ cup sesame seeds
3 tablespoons palm sugar
1 tablespoon coconut oil

MARINADE

big bunch of cilantro, finely chopped, plus more for serving
¼ cup sesame oil
⅓ cup soy sauce
1 tablespoon sambal oelek or Sriracha
3 garlic cloves, finely chopped to a paste
1 tablespoon freshly grated ginger
1 tablespoon tamarind paste
1 teaspoon salt

Tempura with Wasabi Mayo Dip

OVEN-BAKED VEGETABLES IN CHICKPEA BATTER

This crunchy dish is inspired by Indian pakoras and Japanese tempura—both battered, deep-fried vegetables. In this recipe the vegetables are baked for a lighter but still crispy texture. I'm using chickpea flour, making this dish both gluten-free (if you use gluten-free bread crumbs) and rich in protein. Serve these delicious oven-roasted vegetables as a starter, side dish, or snack.

Preheat the oven to 400°F and line a baking sheet with parchment. Peel and clean the mixed vegetables as needed. Cut any chunky vegetables, such as sweet potato, into sticks or wedges.

Mix the batter ingredients in a bowl and spread the panko on a plate. Dip the vegetables first in the batter to coat, then roll them in panko. Transfer to the baking sheet and bake for 10 to 15 minutes, or until the vegetables are crisp and golden. Keep an eye on the oven during the last 5 minutes to ensure the vegetables don't burn.

Meanwhile, make the wasabi mayo dip by whisking the ingredients until smooth. Serve the battered vegetables with the wasabi dip, hot sauce, and lime wedges.

VE *Use Vegenaise instead of mayonnaise and vegan crème fraîche (page 52) for crème fraîche.*

GF *Use gluten-free bread crumbs.*

SERVES 6 AS A STARTER, SIDE DISH, OR SNACK

2–3 lbs. mixed vegetables, such as kale, sweet potato, onion, broccoli, zucchini blossoms, and green beans

3 cups panko or fine bread crumbs

BATTER

2¼ cups chickpea flour
½ cup water
¾ teaspoon salt
1 teaspoon paprika
1 teaspoon red pepper flakes

WASABI MAYO DIP

1 tablespoon wasabi paste
½ cup mayonnaise
½ cup crème fraîche
salt

FOR SERVING

hot sauce
lime wedges

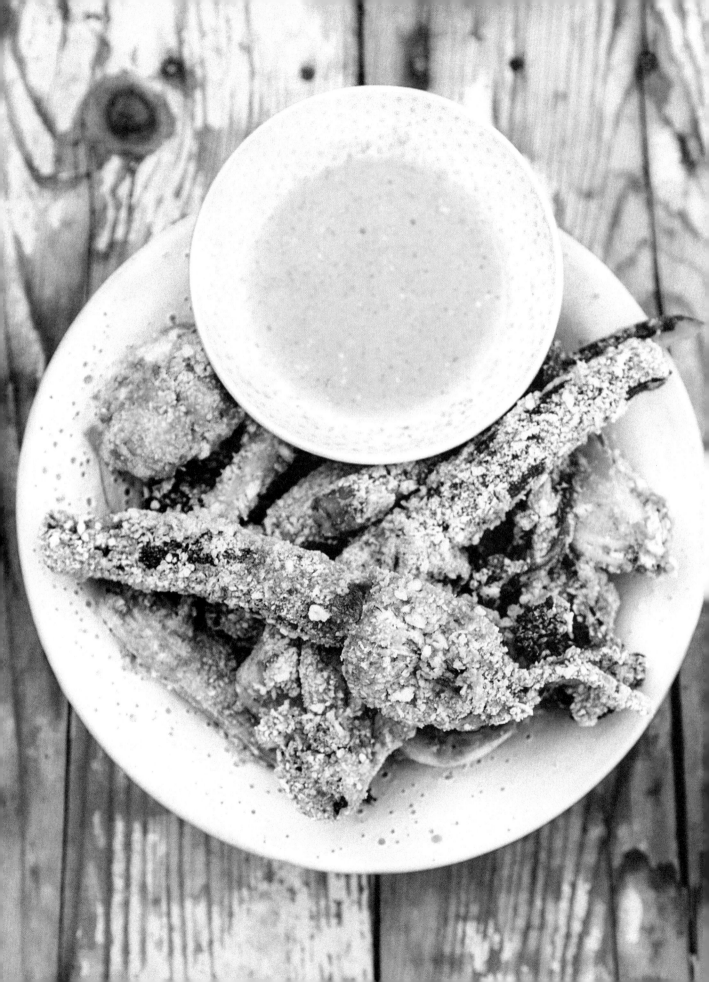

Zoodles on the Side

ZUCCHINI NOODLES WITH TOASTED PINE NUTS AND GREEN TAHINI DRESSING

Cold zoodles make a great side salad for a buffet, offering a cool contrast to warm grilled dishes. In particular, they are a great partner to neatballs (see page 164)! The sauce is a tahini version of a green goddess dressing with plenty of herbs. If you like, spike it with a teaspoon of chlorella for added goodness. Add the dressing just before serving to prevent the zoodles from getting soggy.

SERVES 6 TO 8 AS A SIDE DISH
2 zucchini, spiralized
big bunch of arugula
2–3 handfuls of pine nuts

GREEN TAHINI DRESSING
¼ cup tahini
2 garlic cloves, finely chopped
    to a paste
3 tablespoons almond butter
¼ cup olive oil
juice of 1 lemon
handful of parsley, finely chopped
handful of basil, finely chopped
1 teaspoon chlorella powder
    (optional)
salt and pepper

Blend the dressing ingredients into a smooth sauce.

Heat a skillet and toast the pine nuts until fragrant and golden.

Mix the zoodles with the arugula and toasted pine nuts. Serve with the green tahini dressing.

VE ✓ GF ✓

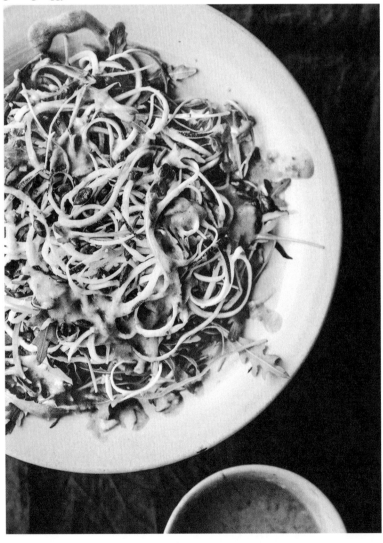

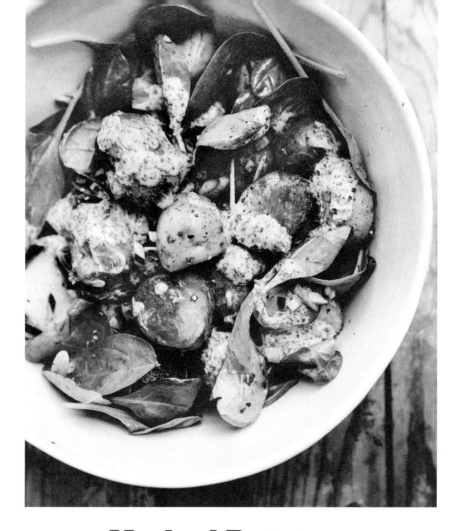

Herbed Potatoes

ROASTED BABY POTATOES WITH CHIVE AND DILL PESTO SAUCE

Baby potatoes with a chive and dill pesto tastes like a Nordic summer. Serve this salad as part of a larger meal, as a filling side dish in a buffet, or with neatballs (see page 164).

Baby potatoes don't need to be peeled and only need a little wash or scrubbing. You can also make this salad with larger potatoes, but scrub or peel the potatoes thoroughly before roasting. Extend the roasting time by 5 to 10 minutes for larger potatoes.

Preheat the oven to 425°F. Spread the potato halves on a baking sheet, drizzle with olive oil, and sprinkle with a little salt and pepper. Roast the potatoes, turning occasionally, until tender and golden brown, about 20 minutes. Watch the potatoes in the last 5 minutes to avoid burning.

Meanwhile, blend the pesto ingredients to a fine loose paste. Remove the potatoes from the oven and place in a big serving bowl. Add the baby spinach and sprinkle with red onions and pine nuts. Drizzle with half the pesto sauce and toss everything to coat. Serve with the rest of the pesto sauce.

VE *Serve with vegan crème fraîche and rawmesan instead of Parmesan.*

GF ✓

SERVES 4

2 lbs. fresh potatoes, halved and scrubbed
olive oil
salt and pepper
2 cups baby spinach
¹/₂ red onion, diced
handful of pine nuts

CHIVE AND DILL PESTO SAUCE

1 garlic clove
2 handfuls of chives
handful of fresh dill
handful of parsley
¹/₄ cup crème fraîche (optional)
3 tablespoons extra-virgin olive oil
1 tablespoon Parmesan or nutritional yeast
juice of 1 lemon
salt and pepper

Neatballs

UNIVERSAL VEGGIE BALLS FLAVORED BY UMAMI POTION

There are no longer any excuses for sad veggie balls. These are made using an umami potion to create a powerful flavor that will have you coming back for more! And they are just as good in a tomato sauce as they are in a masala (see page 140). You can use this as your basic recipe for all kinds of veggie neatballs. Customize the flavor by adding your choice of spice blend, such as taco spices for Mexican or ras el hanout or harissa for North African. They are the perfect party food but also make a lovely addition to a weeknight pasta (see page 120).

Mix the ingredients for the umami potion in a small bowl.

Mix the oats, salt, oregano, and nutritional yeast or Parmesan in a large bowl. Add the rice and pine nuts and mix well.

Heat a skillet over medium-high heat. Add a drizzle of olive oil and cook the onion, mushrooms, and tarragon for 5 minutes, stirring. Transfer to the bowl with the rice mix. Add the carrot, scallions, and parsley to the bowl and mix everything thoroughly with a spoon. Pour the umami potion over the mixture and work it in with a fork. Season with salt and pepper to taste.

Roll the mixture into small balls using the palms of your hands. If the mix is too wet, add a little more dry oats. Roll the balls in panko or bread crumbs.

Heat a skillet over medium-high heat. Add a drizzle of olive oil to the pan and fry the neatballs for a couple of minutes to get a lovely browned surface (you may need to fry in batches, so keep the first batch warm in the oven on its lowest setting). You can turn up the heat for the last minute to get a crisper crust. Add more cooking oil as needed. Remove from the heat, lightly salt, and serve immediately.

VE ✓

GF *Choose gluten-free panko or bread crumbs. Use gluten-free tamari instead of soy sauce. Check your oast are certified free from gluten contamination.*

MAKES 30, SERVING 4

2½ cups ground (Scottish style) oatmeal, plus extra if needed
¾ teaspoon salt
1 teaspoon chopped oregano leaves
2 tablespoons nutritional yeast or Parmesan
1½ cups cooked brown rice
¾ cup pine nuts, ground fine
olive oil
1 red onion, finely minced
¾ lb. mushrooms, chopped
1½ tablespoons chopped tarragon leaves
1 small carrot or ½ large one, finely grated
2 scallions, finely chopped
handful of finely chopped parsley
4 cups panko or fine bread crumbs

UMAMI POTION

1 tablespoon tahini
3 tablespoons soy sauce
2 tablespoons olive oil
1 tablespoon water
juice of ½ lemon
1 teaspoon maple syrup
1 tablespoon Sriracha
1 teaspoon fennel seeds, ground
3 garlic cloves, finely chopped to a paste
1 teaspoon liquid smoke

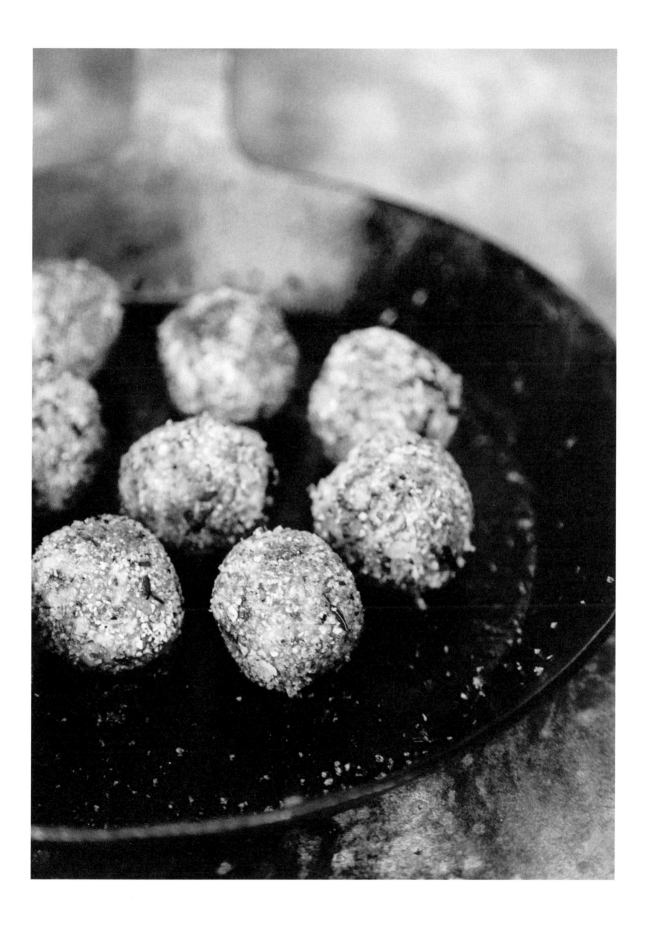

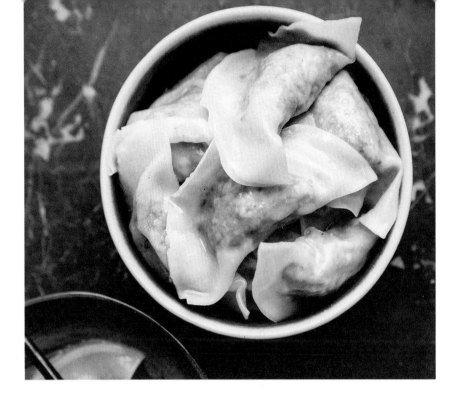

Shiitake and Tofu Dumplings

LITTLE BAGS OF UMAMI-FLAVORED GOODNESS WITH A SWEET AND SOUR DIPPING SAUCE

Dumplings are easy and really delicious. These with tofu, mushrooms, and seaweed make great party food. Make double or triple the quantity for a bigger gathering. I'm using seaweed here as it adds a lovely seafood taste but avoid the extra salted variety. Serve with the sweet and sour dipping sauce.

Pulse the dumpling filling in a food processor, but stop before it becomes too smooth. You want to break it up but not make a purée.

To make the dumpling dough, mix a small amount of flour and water in a bowl, knead, and then add the rest of the water and flour bit by bit. Continue kneading for a few minutes until the dough is not sticky. Cover with a damp dishtowel and refrigerate for 30 minutes.

Knead the dough, then cut it into 4 equal pieces. Roll each piece into a long rope and cut each rope into 10 pieces, making 40 dumpling wrappers. Roll each piece out to a paper-thin circle.

With a moistened fingertip, dampen the edges of a wrapper with water. Place a tablespoon of the filling in the middle of the wrapper, close the wrapper by folding over and press the edges between your thumb and index finger. You can also seal it by making pleats or a little wrap.

Keep the filled dumplings under a damp dishtowel until ready to fry them to keep them from drying out.

Add a little vegetable oil to a skillet and fry the dumplings for 30 seconds, then add a generous splash of water and cover immediately. Steam for 3 minutes. Fry and steam in batches. Serve with the dipping sauce.

Tip! Use ready-made dumpling wrappers!

VE ✓ **GF** *This recipe is not gluten-free.*

40 DUMPLINGS

DUMPLING DOUGH
2 cups wheat flour
³/₄ cup water

FILLING
³/₄ lb. shiitake mushrooms, chopped
    and sautéed for 4 minutes
12 oz. smoked tofu, diced small
handful of dulse seaweed, soaked
    for 30 minutes, drained, and
    chopped (optional)
2 carrots, diced small
8 scallions, finely chopped
1 cup finely chopped white or
    Chinese cabbage
drizzle of soy sauce
2 garlic cloves, finely chopped
    to a paste
1 teaspoon freshly grated ginger

DIPPING SAUCE
1 tablespoon toasted sesame oil
¹/₄ cup rice vinegar
¹/₄ cup water
1 teaspoon honey or agave syrup
¹/₄ teaspoon grated ginger (optional)
pinch of red pepper flakes

Basic Pickles

THEY ADD TANG AND INTEREST TO YOUR BOWLS

Pickles are one of those foods that I make sure I always keep in the fridge as they are universally good and add edge and finish to everything from salads and stir-fries to comforting stews and sandwiches. Making your own pickles is done in a flash! Just drizzle vinegar and add flavorings if you like. A little bit of sweetness elevates the pickles to a dreamy level. Here are a few of my favorites that work with a variety of dishes.

Use sterilized jars and add your chosen pickle ingredients. Seal with a lid and store in the fridge for up to 3 weeks.

VE ✓ GF ✓

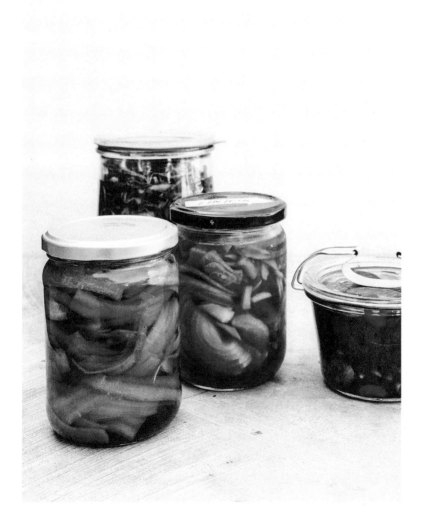

4 QUICKLY PICKLED JARS

QUICK RED ONION PICKLE
  (makes a medium-small jar)
¼ cup apple cider vinegar
⅔ cup water
1 teaspoon salt
½ tablespoon sugar
1 red onion, sliced

INDIAN CARROT
  (makes a medium jar)
2–3 carrots, shaved into thin bands
½ cup rice vinegar
⅔ cup water
juice of 1 lime
1 teaspoon freshly grated ginger
½ teaspoon sugar

PICKLED BEETS
  (makes a small jar)
1 beet, peeled and cut into
  thin wedges
1 shallot, diced
¼ cup red wine vinegar
⅔ cup water
1 tablespoon sugar

SPICY CABBAGE AND
  SEAWEED PICKLE
  (makes a big jar)
¼ small red cabbage, shredded
handful of seaweed (dulse, seaweed
  spaghetti, or wakame)
1–2 carrots, shredded
½ cup rice vinegar
1 cup water
3 garlic cloves, crushed
1 tablespoon freshly grated ginger
handful of toasted sesame seeds
1 apple
¾ teaspoon salt
2 tablespoons Gochujang (or red
  pepper flakes)

Fennel Purée

SILKY FENNEL MASH FOR EVERYDAY MEALS OR DINNER PARTIES

Mashes are delicious with fried and crispy additions, such as the neatballs or any sautéed or roasted vegetables. This delicious mash can be made with a base of potato or Jerusalem artichokes, but it's the fennel that adds interest and makes this mash special. This purée is perfect when you're hosting and want a fancier alternative to regular mashed potatoes.

Cook the potato and fennel in the broth for 15 minutes, or until tender. Drain but reserve a little cooking liquid. Mash the potato and fennel until smooth, using the leftover broth to achieve desired consistency. Season with salt and pepper to taste and serve with a drizzle of extra-virgin olive oil.

Tip! Serve with neatballs (see page 164) and pesto sauce (see page 120).

SERVES 8 AS SIDE DISH
1–2 lbs. potatoes or Jerusalem artichokes, cut into pieces
½ lb. fennel (about half a bulb), cut into pieces
4 cups vegetable broth (see page 56)
salt and pepper
extra-virgin olive oil

VE ✓ GF ✓

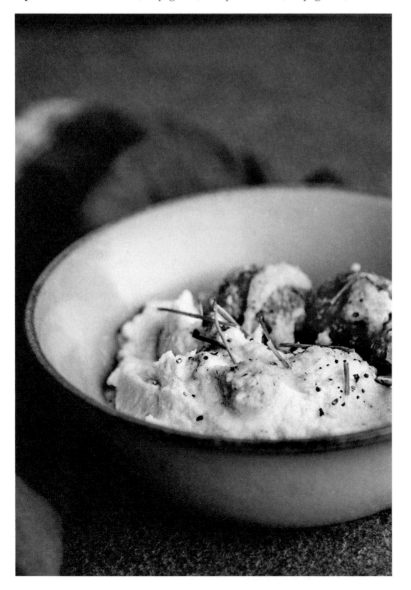

MASH IT UP! *Steaming is one of the best ways to preserve nutrition in cooked vegetables. For nourishing meals, steam vegetables and blend them into a delicious purée. It's a perfect side dish. Almost all vegetables can be mashed, but not all stay firm like potatoes. A tip is to add cooked potatoes if your purée is too loose. Cauliflower and broccoli are delicious to mash and all root vegetables are great in mash.*

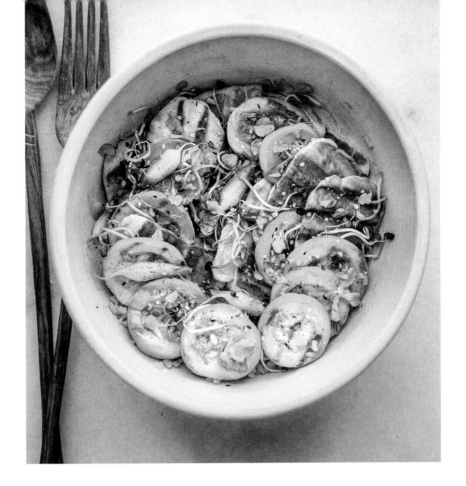

Grilled Halloumi and Zucchini

SALTY MIDDLE EASTERN CHEESE AND JUICY ZUCCHINI SALAD

Grilled halloumi is a fantastic addition to a vegetarian buffet where it makes a great counterpart to fresh, juicy vegetables, salads, and cooked grains. In particular, I like to balance its saltiness by layering it with sweet, grilled zucchini. For a festive look and interesting flavor addition, top with pink radishes, radish sprouts, and edible flowers. You can serve this with the tabbouleh on page 152 as your cooked grain.

Mix the dressing and set aside. Heat a grill pan. Add a drizzle of olive oil and grill the zucchini on both sides until golden with grill marks.

Wipe out the grill pan and reheat, then add the halloumi and grill on both sides until crisp and golden.

Layer the zucchini and halloumi in a bowl, and add your chosen toppings. Drizzle with a few spoons of the dressing and offer the rest on the side. Serve with grains for a full meal or without as an addition to a buffet.

VE *Use tempeh instead of halloumi.*
GF *Serve with a gluten-free grain.*

SERVES 6 TO 8
1 yellow zucchini, cut in ¼-inch
    slices
1 lb. halloumi, cut in ¼-inch slices
salt and pepper
serve with cooked rice, tabbouleh,
    freekeh, or bulgur (see page 152)

DRESSING
1 garlic clove, finely chopped
    to a paste
1 tablespoon agave syrup
¼ cup olive oil, plus more for
    grilling
juice of 2 lemons
pinch of red pepper flakes

TOPPINGS
handful of baby radishes
handful of edible viola or other
    pink flowers
handful of hemp seeds
radish sprouts

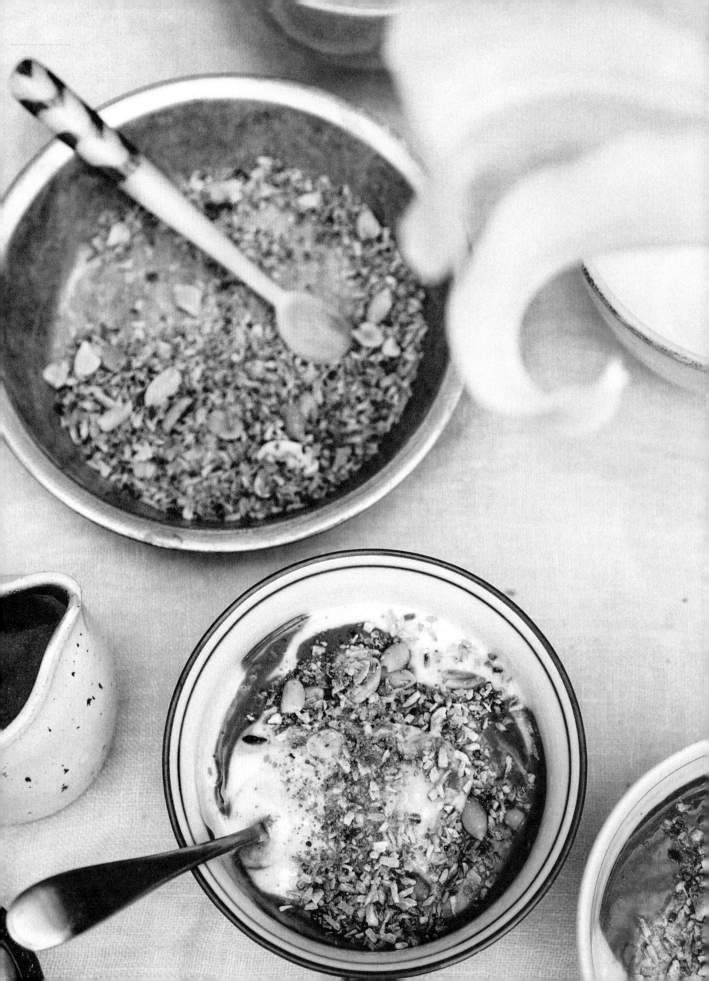

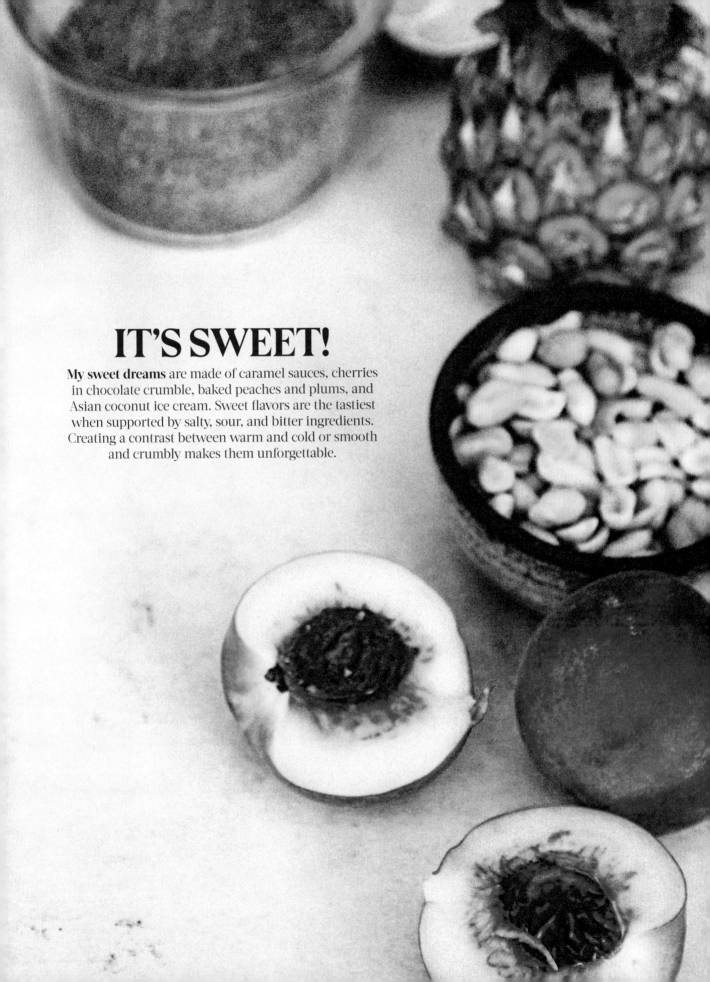

IT'S SWEET!

My sweet dreams are made of caramel sauces, cherries in chocolate crumble, baked peaches and plums, and Asian coconut ice cream. Sweet flavors are the tastiest when supported by salty, sour, and bitter ingredients. Creating a contrast between warm and cold or smooth and crumbly makes them unforgettable.

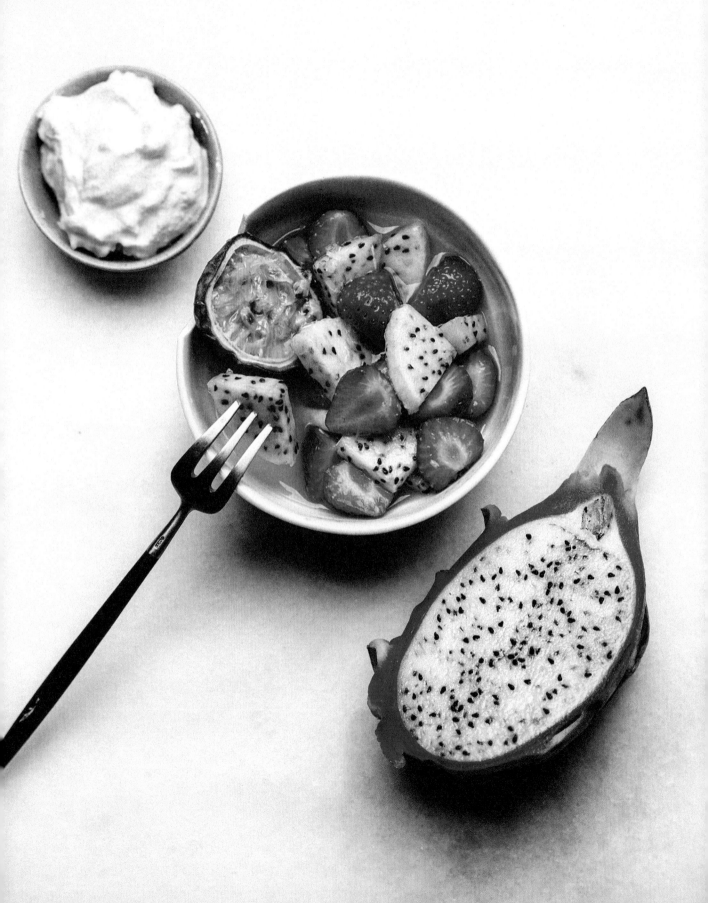

Tropical Fruit with Lime and Lemongrass

FRESH DRAGON FRUIT, PAPAYA, AND STRAWBERRIES WITH TANGY DRESSING

I love a fresh fruit salad in the summer. It's cooling and so easy to make. Using tropical fruit and a tangy lime and lemongrass dressing is an interesting twist on the classic version and brings a touch of paradise in hot weather, the zesty dressing elevating the fruit to new heights. This recipe is a pick-me-up fruit boost and is great to serve to guests. It's the dressing that's key, so feel free to mix and match any tropical or regular fruit you have available.

Mix the ingredients for the dressing and refrigerate until ready to serve.

Prepare the fruit and toss in a large bowl. Serve with the dressing and ice cream, decorated with edible flowers. Coconut ice cream is a dream here but a regular vanilla nice or ice cream is a good fit, too.

VE *Serve with vegan ice cream.*
GF ✓

SERVES 4

1 dragon fruit (pitaya), trimmed and cut into roughly ¹/₂-inch triangles
4 passion fruits, halved
³/₄ cup strawberries, hulled and halved
2 kiwi, peeled and cut into roughly 1-inch triangles
10–12 golden berries

LIME AND LEMONGRASS DRESSING
zest and juice of 2 limes
¹/₄ teaspoon freshly grated ginger
1 lemongrass stalk, inner soft part only, finely chopped
1¹/₂ tablespoon agave or maple syrup
3 tablespoons water

TO SERVE
coconut ice cream (see page 187), coconut yogurt, mascarpone, or another cool, creamy addition of your choice
edible flowers

Peaches and Plums

BAKED STONE FRUIT, PEARS, AND RASPBERRIES WITH OAT CRUMBLES

This recipe is a beautiful balance of flavors and textures, the nutty crunch of the crumble contrasting with the softness of the stone fruit, raspberries, and sweet pear juices. The tangy orange and herbal aromas of the rosemary add interest and a feeling that it's coming straight out of Grandma's oven. Comforting, delicious, and intriguing. This crumble is both easier and more juicy than a fruit pie, with the added bonus of also being lighter.

Preheat the oven to 400°F. Combine the crumble ingredients in a bowl. Arrange the prepared peaches, plums, and pears in a baking dish with the raspberries. Sprinkle with coconut sugar and orange zest and tuck in the rosemary. Drizzle with the orange juice, maple syrup, and vanilla extract. Toss to coat, then bake for 15 minutes. Remove from the oven, scatter the crumble loosely over the top and return to the oven for 5 to 7 minutes.

Divide between four serving bowls. Serve with mascarpone, ice cream, or cashew cream.

VE *Serve with cashew cream or vegan nice cream.*

GF *Check that your oats are certified free from gluten contamination.*

SERVES 4

4–5 peaches, halved and pitted
4–5 plums, halved and pitted
2 pears, halved and cored
³/₄ cup raspberries
3 tablespoons coconut sugar
zest and juice of 1 unwaxed orange
sprig of rosemary
3 tablespoons maple syrup
¹/₂ teaspoon vanilla extract

CRUMBLE

3 tablespoons melted coconut oil
   or olive oil
2 tablespoons palm sugar
handful of finely chopped
   hazelnuts
2 handfuls of oats
¹/₂ cup shredded coconut
pinch of salt

TO SERVE

mascarpone, ice cream, or
   cashew cream

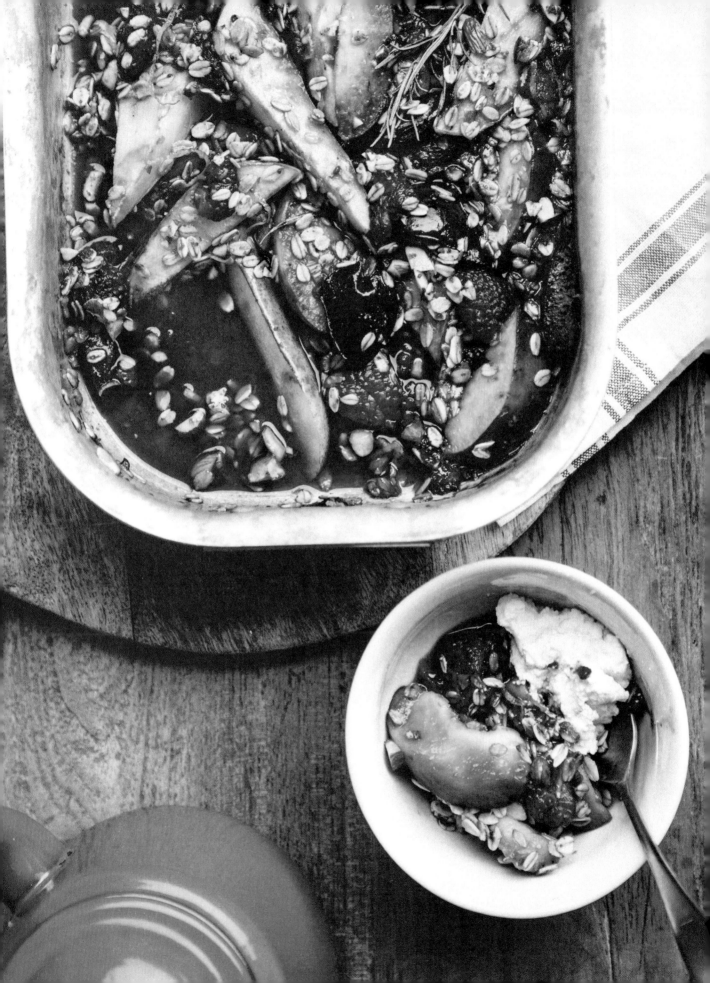

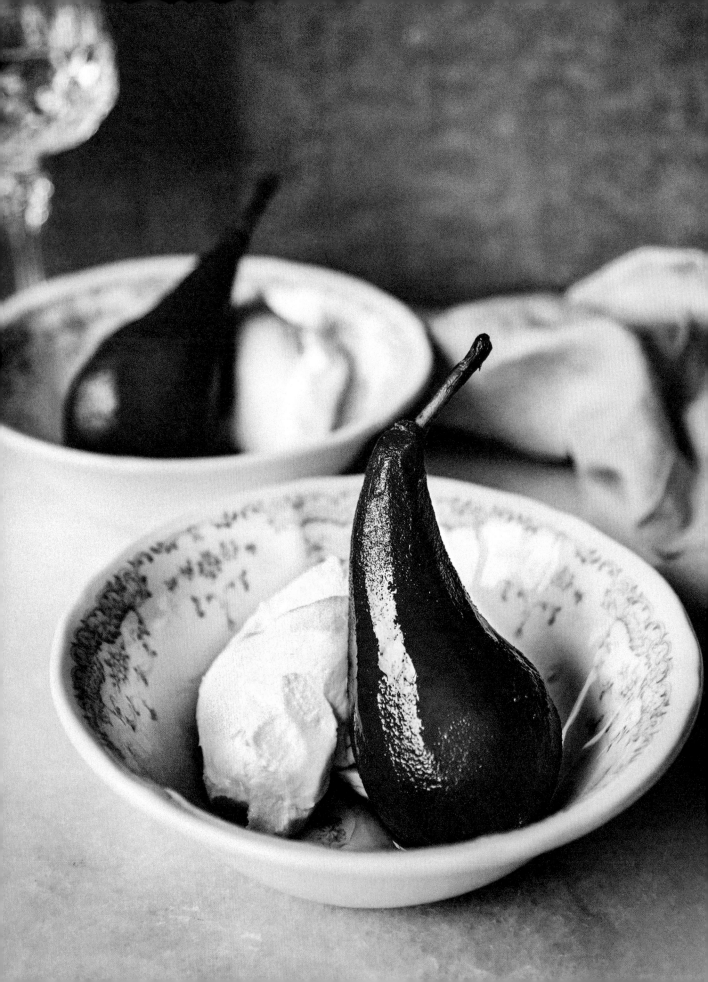

Chai Vanilla Pears

PEARS POACHED IN CHAI AND RED WINE

Poached pears are impressive when you have guests and in this recipe they take on an extra dimension by being infused with chai tea spices. Also called chai masalas, these originate from India where chai tea has been a popular herbal remedy since the days when the ancient Ayurvedic scriptures were penned. The typical Indian flavors used in a chai blend—cardamom, ginger, black tea, and cloves—are popular in Northern European mulled wine. This grown-up dessert is especially lovely in the autumn and winter months and you can easily use apples instead of pears.

Peel the pears carefully, place in a saucepan with the wine and vanilla, and add water to cover. Bring to a boil, then turn down the heat to a simmer. Add the tea bags and infuse for 3 minutes, then remove them from the pan. Cover and continue to simmer the pears over low heat for 30 minutes.

Remove the pears from the liquid. Serve with mascarpone, orange zest, and a drizzle of maple syrup.

VE *Omit the mascarpone.*
GF ✓

SERVES 4
4 ripe and firm bosc pears
$1\frac{1}{2}$ cups red wine
1 teaspoon vanilla extract
2 chai tea bags

TO SERVE
1 lb. mascarpone
orange zest
maple or agave syrup

Nice Cream and Caramel Sauce

FROZEN BANANA NICE CREAM WITH ALMOND CARAMEL SAUCE, COCONUT, AND PEANUT

There are three brilliant things in this recipe. First, banana nice cream is fabulous: it uses only one ingredient—frozen banana! Just process to a smooth consistency and it's ready to go. Second, the combination of toasted coconut and peanuts is rarely bettered—its nutty sweetness elevates stir-fries, sandwiches, salads, and, yes . . . ice cream! And, last but not least, the caramel sauce can be added to various desserts and fruits for that perfect hit of sweet-meets-savory. Natural sweetness at its best.

Blend the ingredients for the almond caramel sauce in a food processor or blender until smooth.

To make the coconut and peanut shred, put shredded coconut and peanuts in a food processor and pulse for a few seconds. It should be a rough mixture with the peanuts broken up. Heat a skillet and toast the mixture, then let cool.

Put the bananas in a food processor and pulse until they are an ice cream consistency. Serve the nice cream topped with the coconut shred and almond caramel sauce.

VE ✓ GF ✓

SERVES 4

ALMOND CARAMEL SAUCE
$\frac{1}{2}$ cup coconut sugar
$\frac{1}{2}$ cup almond milk
drizzle of neutral-flavored
   vegetable oil
2 tablespoons almond butter
   (optional)
pinch of salt

COCONUT AND PEANUT SHRED
2 cups shredded coconut
$\frac{1}{2}$ cup peanuts

NICE CREAM
8 bananas, frozen in pieces

GOING BANANAS WITH NICE CREAM
Make different flavored nice creams by adding ingredients like fruit and berries, cacao, or matcha powder. The natural sweetness of bananas means you don't need to add any sweetener to the nice cream. The riper the banana is, the better for nice-cream making, so don't throw away bananas that are turning brown. Freeze them and make delicious nice cream instead.

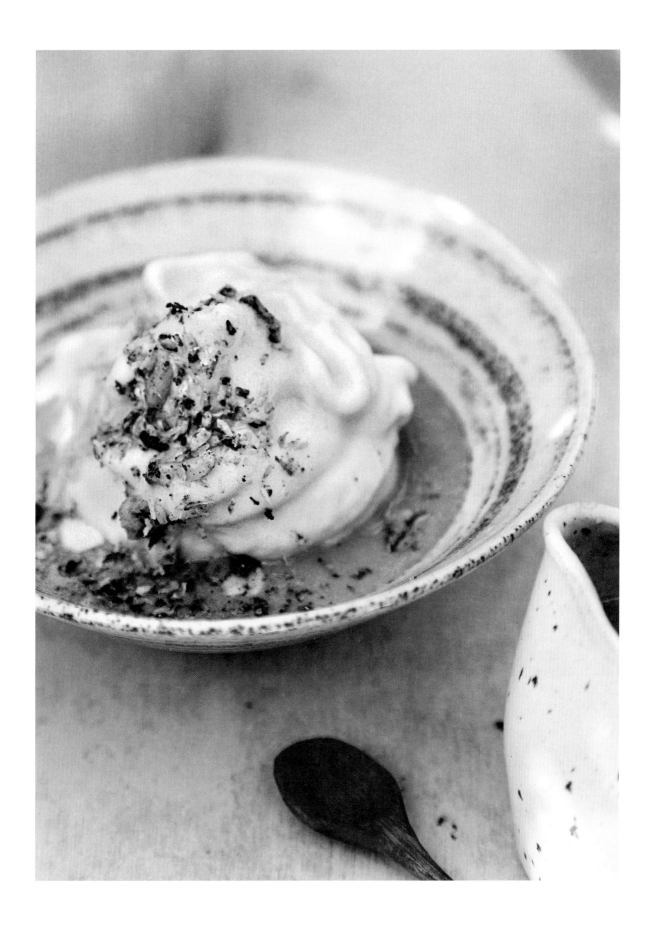

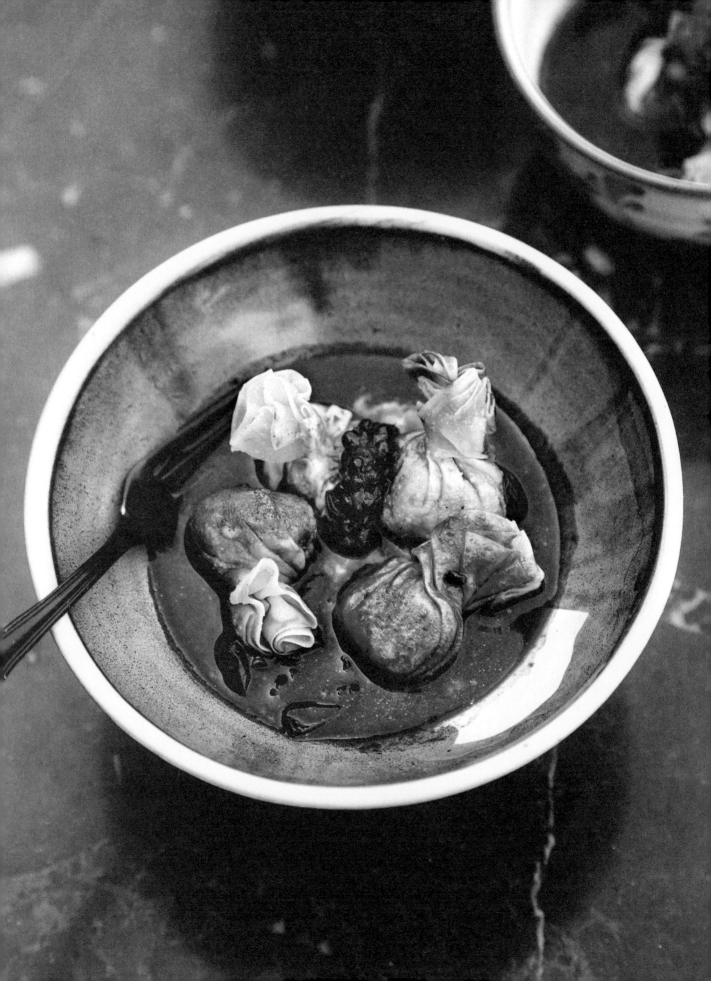

Orange Almond Dumplings in Blackberry Soup

TANGY COCONUT AND ALMOND DUMPLINGS WITH BLACKBERRIES

These dumplings are filled with a zesty orange–almond paste and served in a sweet blackberry sauce. They're great when you have guests as everything can be prepared beforehand, and the dumplings cooked just before serving. If you like, you can add a spoonful of creamy ricotta or cottage cheese, but they're just as lovely without it.

I use the ready-made dumpling wrappers found in Asian supermarkets and well-stocked food stores.

Add the blackberry sauce ingredients to a saucepan over medium-high heat and simmer for 5 minutes. Remove from heat and let it cool, then transfer to a food processor. Blend until smooth, then refrigerate.

To make the filling, blend the ingredients into a smooth paste.

Place a dumpling wrapper on your work surface and add a teaspoon of the filling in the middle of the wrapper. Moisten the edges of the wrapper with water, then fold the edges over the filling, making pleats as you close and seal the dumplings between your fingertips. Continue with the rest of the wrappers until you have used all of the filling.

Heat a skillet over medium heat and add a drizzle of vegetable oil. Make sure the surface of the pan is well coated, then place the dumplings in the pan so they don't touch, in batches if necessary. Cook the dumplings for 2 to 3 minutes over medium-low heat. Remove from the pan and serve with the blackberry sauce and ricotta.

VE *This recipe is vegan if you omit ricotta or cottage cheese. Or serve with a spoonful of vegan crème fraîche (see page 50).*

GF *Buy gluten-free dumpling wrappers.*

SERVES 4 (5 DUMPLINGS
 PER PERSON)
20 ready-made dumpling wrappers
 (plus a few extra for practicing
 your folds), or make your own
 dough (recipe on page 166)
neutral-flavored vegetable oil
ricotta, for serving

BLACKBERRY SAUCE
4–5 cups blackberries
²/₃ cup water
juice of ½ lemon
¼ cup palm sugar
1 tablespoon maple syrup

FILLING
2 handfuls toasted almonds
 or pistachios
1 teaspoon vanilla extract
2 tablespoons orange juice
1 tablespoon coconut oil
¾ cup desiccated coconut
pinch of salt
2 tablespoons agave syrup

Cherry Choco and Sea Salt Crumble

STOVETOP CRUMBLE WITH SALTED COCONUT CREAM

I love baking but sometimes my cravings want a quicker fix, hence the invention of stovetop cookie-like crumble treats such as this one. It is perfect with whipped coconut cream.

To make the coconut whip, combine the chilled coconut cream with salt, lemon juice, and sugar in a mixing bowl and whip to a fluffy cream with an electric mixer. Keep covered in the fridge until ready to serve and whip up again if needed.

Mix the choco granola ingredients in a bowl. Heat a skillet and toast the crumble over medium-low heat (in batches if needed) until the crumble is crisp and fragrant, about 2 to 3 minutes.

Serve with the coconut whip or any other cool creamy addition like mascarpone or yogurt, and top with the cherries or berries.

VE *Use vegan creme fraiche or soygurt instead of mascarpone. Choose vegan ice cream.*

GF *Use certified gluten-free oat flakes instead of spelt flakes.*

SERVES 4

COCONUT WHIP
(can be replaced with dairy whipped cream)
14 oz. can coconut cream, chilled overnight
pinch of salt
2 tablespoons sugar of your choice
squeeze of lemon juice

CHOCO GRANOLA
3 cups spelt flakes or oat flakes
1/4 cup olive oil
1 1/2 cups desiccated coconut
2 1/2 tablespoons raw cacao powder (or cocoa powder)
1/2 teaspoon vanilla extract
1/4 cup palm sugar
3/4 cup almonds or pistachios
pinch of salt

TO SERVE
mascarpone or ice cream (if not making the coconut whip)
cherries or blueberries

KEEPING IT COOL: *To make coconut whipped cream, buy a can of coconut cream or full-fat coconut milk and chill overnight. Don't shake the can as it disrupts the thickening and hardening.*

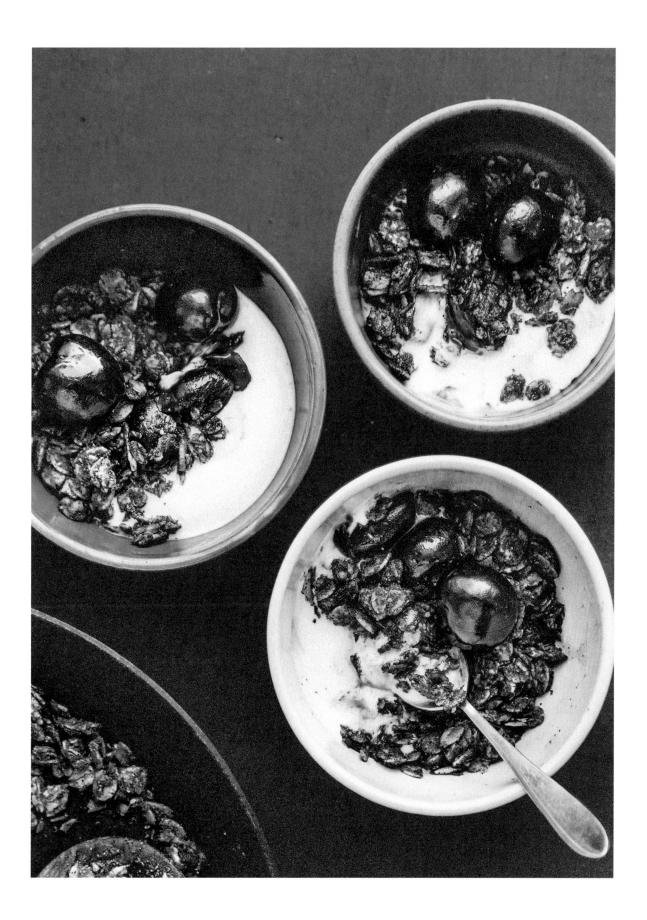

Cashew Chocolate Cream

RAW CACAO, MEDJOOL DATES, AND CASHEW PUDDING

This sinfully good vegan chocolate mousse is really easy to make. If you soak cashews for a couple of hours or overnight all you need to do is to transfer the ingredients to a blender, push the button, and let it do the magic. For sweetness, I use medjool dates—a popular choice for whole-food cooking. They add a delicious sweetness with hints of caramel. Avocado lends a buttery smoothness to the mousse.

VE ✓ GF ✓

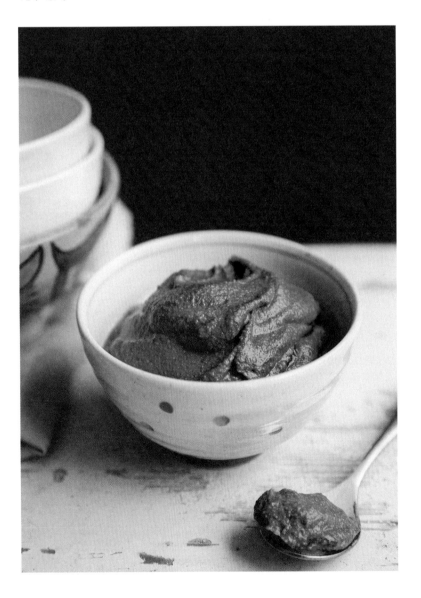

SERVES 2 TO 4

2 cups cashews, soaked overnight and drained
1 avocado, pitted, peeled, and cut into pieces
6 tablespoons raw cacao powder
1/2 teaspoon vanilla extract
2 tablespoons coconut oil
1 cup nut milk
8 medjool dates, pitted and roughly chopped
pinch of salt

SUGGESTED STIR-INS

1 tablespoon orange juice and 1 tablespoon orange zest
handful of toasted hazelnuts for a nutella flavor
pinch of cayenne pepper
1/2 teaspoon lavender extract for a floral taste
1/4 cup espresso for a coffee kick
1/2 teaspoon ground star anise

Blend all the ingredients into a smooth mousse. Divide in bowls.

FAIRTRADE CHOCOLATE!
Our love and demand for chocolate is bringing work and income opportunities to communities in Third World countries. Unfortunately, a great number of people are working with low wages and in inhumane conditions to supply us with our favorite treats and child labor is not uncommon. Support equality by buying Fairtrade branded products of raw cacao, cocoa, and chocolate.

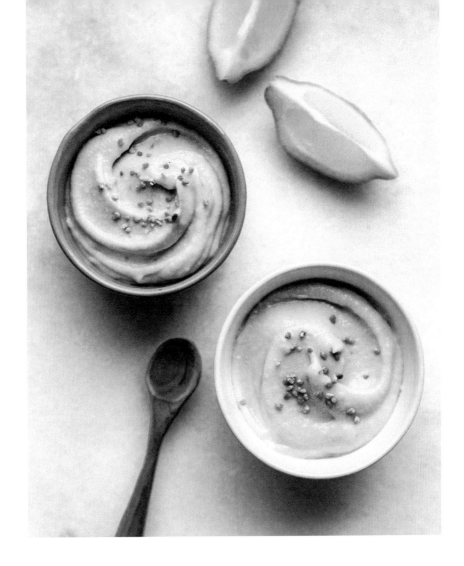

Key Lime Cream

LIME, AVOCADO, AND CASHEW CREAM

Key lime cream is the filling used in Florida's famous Key Lime Pie, but you don't need Florida's locally grown limes or a pie crust to enjoy the best of this pie—the filling. It makes a perfect dessert on its own. Sweet flavors are enhanced by balancing tangy tartness and a tiny bit of saltiness. I absolutely love a little lemon or lime with my sweet treats. Green, cool, and delicious, this refreshing dessert is perfect served chilled in hot weather.

Blend all the ingredients together. Cover and refrigerate for 30 minutes. Serve in bowls.

VE ✓ GF ✓

SERVES 2

1 avocado, pitted and peeled
¾ cup cashews, soaked overnight and drained
½ cup creamy coconut milk
½ cup coconut oil
zest of 1 lime
juice of 2 limes
juice of 1 lemon
1 teaspoon vanilla extract
⅓ cup agave syrup
pinch of salt

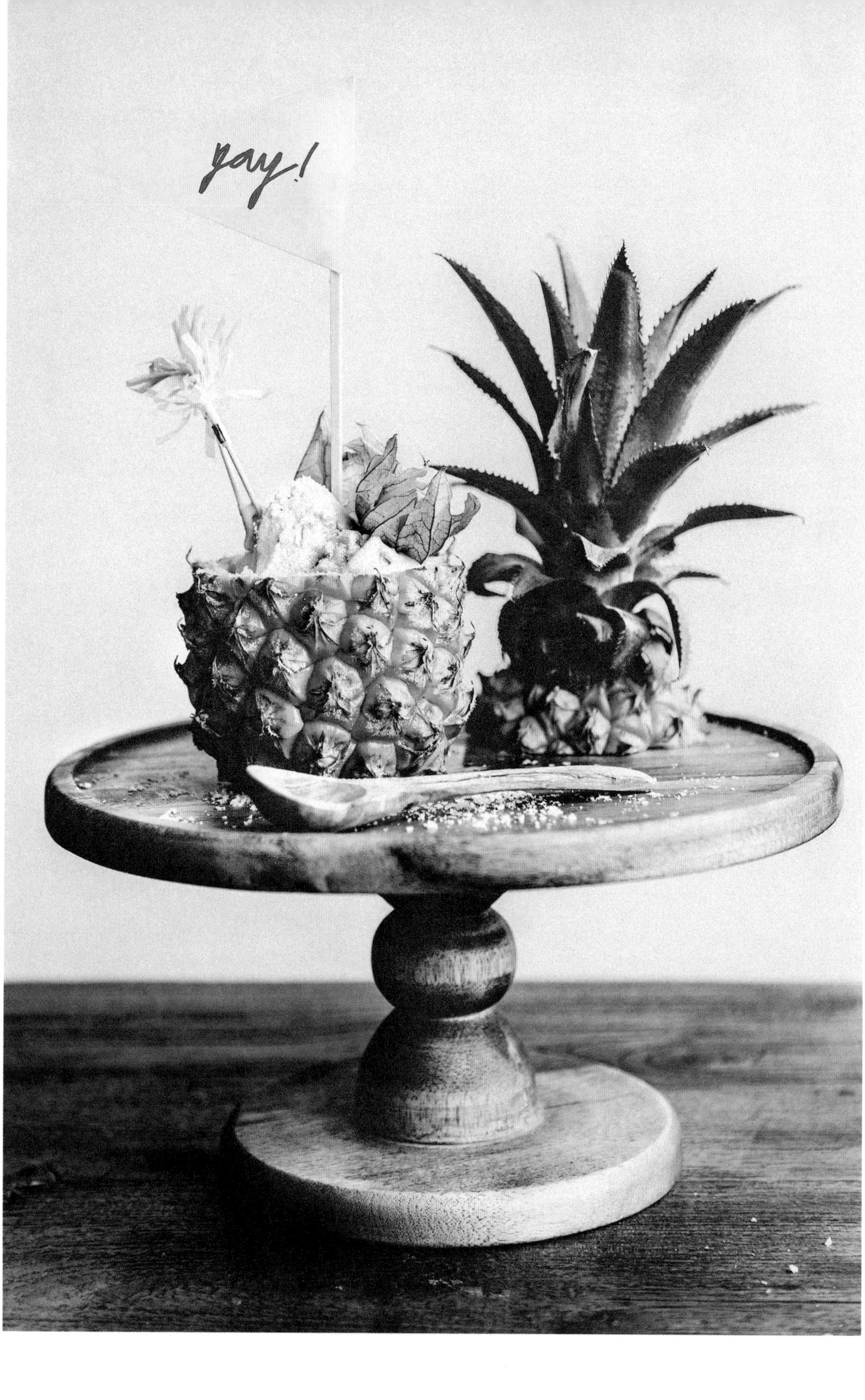
yay!

Coconut Ice Cream

ASIAN-STYLE DAIRY-FREE ICE CREAM

Es krim kelapa! That's the Indonesian name for coconut ice cream, a refreshing, dairy-free dessert that is popular all over Asia. The first time I tasted it, I raved about it for days, it was so good. The basic recipe is the same as for a vanilla ice cream, but you can add a variety of interesting ingredients. Choose only one of the suggested stir-ins, though, if you want to keep a crisp, clean flavor. Add the stir-ins with the rest of the ingredients in the food processor to make versions such as Japanese-style black sesame ice cream or green matcha ice cream.

Blend all the ingredients until smooth in a food processor then pour into a saucepan. Bring to a boil over medium-high heat and cook for 1 to 2 minutes, then remove from the heat.

Pour the mixture into an ice-cream maker and follow the manufacturer's instructions, or freeze in a freezer-proof container for 3 hours, remixing every 30 minutes to break up the ice crystals.

Tip! It's popular to serve coconut ice cream in a coconut shell, but using a hollow fresh pineapple or melon adds a festive and fun touch.

VE ✓ GF ✓

SERVES 4
$\frac{1}{2}$ cup coconut oil, melted
$\frac{1}{2}$ cup agave syrup
$\frac{1}{4}$ cup palm sugar
$3\frac{1}{2}$ cups shredded coconut
2 14 oz. cans coconut milk
pinch of salt
2 teaspoons vanilla extract

STIR-INS (OPTIONAL)
2 handfuls toasted black sesame
  seeds, blended fine
3 tablespoons peanut butter
1 tablespoon fresh lemongrass,
  finely chopped
2 tablespoons raw cacao powder
  and a pinch of cayenne pepper
3 tablespoons espresso
2 tablespoons matcha green
  tea powder
berries and fruit are natural ice
  cream partners—use 1–2 cups
  of chosen berry or fruit

TOPPINGS
fruit or berries of your choice
  (here I used golden berries)

INDEX

Design Resources

Making a cookbook involves a lot of prop styling. I often get asked questions about where I buy my tableware, so I've listed quality providers that I relied on when making this book. Looking for a certain bowl or spoon featured? Visit nourishatelier.com/shopthestyling for more detailed information.

NOY ROAD
Photographer Lina Erikssons's shop, Noy Road, sells beautiful handmade textiles from Southeast Asia. She works closely with craftsmen and -women ensuring the highest quality, fair wages, and natural materials.
www.noyroad.com

SNOEPS
Stylist Silke Feiter makes and sells handmade quality macramé and other craft designs. Her macramé takes time and attention to make, and she also takes customized orders.
www.snoeps.nl

GRAIN AND KNOT
The small, handmade wooden spoons that appear in the book are carved by London-based artist Sophie from Grain and Knot.
www.grainandknot.com

MARGARIDA FERNANDES
Portuguese Margarida makes handmade homeware ceramics that you will love and cherish.
www.margaridamf.com

L'ETOILE CONCEPT STORE
L'etoile Concept Store is a Dutch online shop (you can order from abroad) that sells products made with natural materials for the home and kitchen.
www.letoileconceptstore.nl

SUKHA
Sukha is a concept store with their own brand of homeware and fashion. Sukha work in close collaboration with craftswomen and -men in Nepal.
www.sukha-amsterdam.nl

GAYA CERAMIC
Gaya Ceramic makes stand-out ceramics from their studio in Bali.
www.gayaceramic.com

SPECK AND STONE
Hannah Slade's wood bowls and ceramic pieces are among my absolute favorites.
www.speckandstone.com

VÄSTERGÅRDEN
This Swedish ceramic studio makes customized designs for chefs and restaurants and sells lovely handmade collections through their online shop.
www.vastergarden.se

SISSY BOY
Dutch concept store that sells interior, fashion, and ktichenware. Truly a gem, affordable and full of desirable objects.
www.sissyboy.nl

FALCON ENAMELWARE
I'm a big fan Falcon kitchenware. I never get tired of my cute red teapot, or white-and-blue-rimmed cups.
www.falconenamelware.com

GEKAAPT
Gekaapt sells edgy ceramics, homeware, and fashion. One of the most interesting shops in Amsterdam.
www.gekaapt.nu

STADSPAVILJOEN NOORD
One of my most frequent shopping spots for tableware.
www.stadspaviljoennoord.nl/winkel

PIASTRELLE
Piastrelle sells the finest stone and mosaic.
www.piastrelle.nl

STONE AND MARBLE
Best marble design shop.
www.stonedmarble.com

MOSAIC DEL SUR
Moroccan handmade mosaic, for a dream kitchen.
www.cementtegels.net

FAIR TRADE INTERNATIONAL
Make informed choices. Visit Fair Trade's website to learn more about contributing to a fair global economy.
www.fairtrade.net

THANK YOU

It's said that it takes a village to raise a child! Well you probably heard that authors refer to their book projects as babies. And this book wouldn't have been possible to make without involving a whole bunch of people.

On the top of my list for deserving a big thank you is my family (who are frequent hand models in my shots): Natal, my partner and beloved, for listening, advising, being my handyman and tasting all recipes with me; your honest opinions and loving support mean everything to me. My children, Nova and Evan, for being enthusiastic throughout the making of this book, going out of your way to taste things you were suspicious of and for lending a hand when needed. You are my sunshines! And thank you, mum, for "everything!"
   Thanks to beautiful Gloria for lending yourself to modeling with ease. Nobody holds a bowl more naturally than you! I'd like to thank my friends Suzanne, Jessica, Hans, and Elin for being the most awesome people I know. A sincere "namaste" to my friend and spiritual sister, Leoni Santander, for lending me beautiful ceramics and being a real life inspiration!

Many thanks to my colleagues and friends at *Buffé* magazine in Sweden, especially our editor-in-chief Tony Wallin, for our constant ongoing conversations about culinary trends and obsessions and for taking me to gastronomic experiences at restaurants like Esperanto in Stockholm. You always push me forward and inspire me!

And a warm, big thank you to Sophie, Hannah, and Kyle at Kyle Books for invaluable input, giving me this fantastic opportunity and making this book possible.

I would also like to mention some of the food writers who inspire me. My cooking wouldn't be the same if I had never come across Yotam Ottolenghi's or Jamie Oliver's home-cooked style of food. There's a new wave of vegetarianism growing, and films and books on the subject that truly move me. Jonathan Safran Foer's book *Eating Animals* and the film *Forks Over Knives* have influenced me and my cooking and steered me to a more plant-based diet.
   I'm also a big fan of vegetarian food blogs, such as Sarah Britton's My New Roots, Green Kitchen Stories, Dolly and Oatmeal, and The First Mess. And a number of micro bloggers on Instagram, all sharing a wealth of inspiration on a daily basis. It's all about community, sharing virtual and real-life meals.
   And thank you for buying and reading this book this far. These bowls were made for you.